Alzhe

A Story for Kids of All Ages Who Love Someone

(A Calming Gift for Alzheimer Patients and Senior Citizens Living)

Signe Marshall

Published By **Simon Dough**

Signe Marshall

Alzheimers: A Story for Kids of All Ages Who Love Someone (A Calming Gift for Alzheimer Patients and Senior Citizens Living)

ISBN 978-1-77485-464-8

Legal & Disclaimer

The information contained in this book is not designed to replace or take the place of any form of medicine or professional medical advice. The information in this book has been provided for educational and entertainment purposes only.

The information contained in this book has been compiled from sources deemed reliable, and it is accurate to the best of the Author's knowledge; however, the Author cannot guarantee its accuracy and validity and cannot be held liable for any errors or omissions. Changes are periodically made to this book. You must consult your doctor or get professional medical advice before using any of the suggested remedies, techniques, or information in this book.

TABLE OF CONTENTS

Introduction

If you've received this book, then it's likely that you've loved ones who are suffering from dementia and you're playing the role of caregiver. It's a difficult job to take care of those who are experiencing physical decline and losing the characteristics you may have observed in them. Most often, dementia is associated with troubles with mood, wandering as well as anxiety and confusion, and difficulty communicating. While there may be medications that can help but, in reality, the symptoms can get worse as the condition progresses.

In this book, we aim to offer you some important insight about dementia and the kind of behavior your loved one might display. The following behaviors can be helpful to help you stay at ease and decrease anxiety should a situation occur. The more organized and calm you stay, the better your loved ones will react and this can result in an easier time for them or a less violent or emotional outburst. If you make your home a secure space and making sure that every weakness is addressed and addressed, you will be able to feel confident that your loved one is secure within their home. When it comes to mental and physical activities that you can incorporate your schedule with them, and also, the best ways to make an appropriate and balanced diet You can apply these guidelines to help both of you to adapt to those effects caused by dementia.

There are many books on the subject available out there and I am grateful for picking this one!

Chapter 1: What Is Dementia And How Serious Is It?

The term "dementia" doesn't refer to a specific illness. Instead, it's a broad term that describes the symptoms that can be attributed to an overall decline in memory and cognitive abilities, which can affect the ability of a person to perform their daily activities. In the majority of cases Alzheimer's disease is responsible for more than 80% of cases of dementia, however, there are other types also, depending on how serious your situation is. For instance, vascular dementia may occur following an accident or stroke if a person has difficulty with their cognitive skills and. There are some particular situations where dementia could be easily reversible, like thyroid issues or serious vitamin deficiencies.

There are numerous health conditions which can trigger dementia, but it's crucial to be aware of that it is a sign of the condition. Sometimes, it's portrayed as a normal part of aging, however, it's crucial to understand that memory loss and loss of cognitive capabilities is not normaland is more likely to be a result of an illness known as neurodegenerative. The symptoms of dementia differ greatly and don't necessarily have to be similar for every person. However, the following functions can be affected:

* thinking and judgment skills
* perception of vision
* verbal communication
* Recall and memory
* ability to concentrate on a single task
* Clear thinking

The majority of types of dementia are thought to progress, which means that the symptoms begin at a very slow pace, but begin to worsen with time. It could be an indication of the disease progressing. Research is being carried out to find out how the condition can be passed down through families. Certain forms of dementia can be passed down as an individual gene, but each person has the same set of genes, which can increase or decrease the chances of developing dementia in less obvious ways. Studies on Alzheimer's show that many relatives are infected by this disease in many generations. It could be due to an inheritance of a mutation between parents.

4

Chapter 2: Getting Treatment

There's no single test that can tell whether someone is suffering from dementia and that's the reason it's important to look for clues to the condition of someone. If someone is suffering from mild dementia, like constantly not remembering appointments, or what they store items in or how to complete certain tasks, it's an indication of what might be the start of the process of developing dementia. There are times when other people suffer from memory problems and it doesn't need to be a sign of dementia or be associated to any other illness. If you do notice problems with memory or an abrupt decline in your cognitive abilities The most crucial thing is to see a physician to find out the reason.

An evaluation conducted by a licensed health professional can provide answers about dementia and the degree to which it has advanced. The majority of cases of Alzheimer's are diagnosed through physical examinations, lab tests, mental capabilities, a meticulous medical history examination as well as observing day-to-day functioning behaviors and the ability to recall information. It isn't always easy for medical professionals to identify the kind of dementia because there are many symptoms that can be found in conjunction with. It's possible that you'll need to consult an neurologist or geriatrician to undergo more tests to establish an appropriate treatment plan. A brain scan can reveal the extent to which the condition has advanced.

A quick diagnosis of dementia can aid the person in obtaining treatment or participate in studies or clinical trials to reverse the memory loss. The sooner you recognize it is, the better combat it through exercise and cognitive exercises. Of course, having a diagnosis is crucial to prepare to plan for your future. If you're a family member of person who is living on their own it is possible to change the way they live to ensure they're not on their own. If they live with you, it requires some adjustments to ensure their safety at home.

The treatment for dementia is dependent on the root cause. If it's a form of progressive dementia like Alzheimer's disease, there's no cure or treatment that can stop the progression. Unfortunately, the signs of dementia appear to worsen as it comes to patients suffering from

Alzheimer's. However, there are drugs which can help improve the symptoms. It is also possible to use non-drug therapies to help keep patients in their routines and promote new activities. This could improve their memory and recall abilities and motivate them to utilize their cognitive capabilities despite mental decline.

It is possible that the solution to dementia will be found for the next generations. That's why the funding for research and participation in clinical trials is crucial. If you have a loved one who is willing to participate in clinical trials, it is a fantastic method to ensure that the experience of fighting dementia will be utilized for research to aid future patients.

Chapter 3: Common Dementia-Related Behavior

Dementia is a highly individual process that has no two stages of the disease exactly alike. When the disease first begins to manifest it can appear normal and the patient may be able to forget tiny details or words or losing items. They seem to still be themselves and may appear to be "normal" signs of aging. As dementia gets worse, a variety of symptoms appear and can make it difficult for the individual to lead their daily activities.

A few of these actions may include, but aren't included in:

Confusion: It is typically one of the first symptoms of dementia. It starts by your loved one losing the words they are used to hearing, or common information, or experiencing difficulty recalling information that is new to them. At first, the forgetfulness might seem innocent, but as dementia grows, confusion gets more severe. Your loved one might forget they are as well as where they are and in what year. They might also forget about their life and past memories and experiences that they treasured. It can be difficult to overcome Try to be as calm as you possibly can when you gentle speak to your loved one and acknowledge their feelings about their feelings. Sometimes, repeating the truth isn't helpful since they aren't able to remember.

Modifications to eating patterns: Often people suffering from dementia may shed weight due to forgetting to eat, or suddenly alter how they consume food. They may not enjoy food items they used to love or feel overwhelmed or anxious to eat an entire dinner as they did in the past. If this occurs you should make certain that you're feeding your loved ones with foods and beverages that are filling and healthy and keep an check on them to make sure that they're eating. If they're losing excessive weight, make sure to consult your doctor regarding any medication or supplements.

Insufficient hygiene: People suffering from middle-stage dementia lose interest in their appearance, too. In many cases, when they are at home, they won't take the time to clean the hair or change clothes, or take a bath or shower for several days. If you observe a decline in these behaviors and you notice a change, make certain that you are taking the initiative and encourage them to keep going. Set up a routine each of you with your beloved ones take part in together, so that they feel fulfilled. If they seem to have forgotten how help, encourage them to practice and replicate the actions to aid them in remembering.

Sundowning is a term used to describe the hyperactive or anxious behaviour that dementia sufferers display during the evening hours. It is believed that they are exhausted by the many tasks they engage in during the day. When you add that to the confusion in their minds, they could find it difficult to communicate their frustrations or adequately communicate their physical and mental fatigue. To stay clear of this anxious "witching time," try and avoid intense activities like bathing, exercising or eating at this time. Instead, create an hour of peace where the individual can unwind or read the time with their loved ones as they prepare to go to sleeping. Beware of caffeine and sugar during this time as it may just make them more aggressive. Keep calm and calm if mood changes occur and remember that your loved ones need affirmation of their emotions.

Bitterness and Accusations The most calm people can be prone to a series of accusation and a bitter rage as they suffer from dementia. In most cases, they will lashed out at family or caregivers friends and blame them for lying or hiding details from them. They might accuse them of absconding with their possessions or keeping them in a confined space but not permitting them move in the way they once did. Keep in mind that when these changes occur and they're not an criticism of you. It's dementia, not your beloved one. Do not try to argue, instead try to change the subject and divert them to a different topic or activity. Re-direction will be an important tool in dealing with people with dementia since it will assist in preventing the escalation of disagreements.

Hand-Wringingand Pacing, as well as Rocking Back and forth Physical motions like these could be ways that the patient with dementia manifests their anxiety. They may become restless and trigger by any changes in their surroundings, or even new emotions or emotions. If you observe these signs, you should take the time to talk with your loved one and determine the root of the anxiety. Try diverting their attention to ease their anxiety and suggest a relaxing activity like walking and playing music.

Repetition of false stories A loved one may be telling stories that were never true, but which they appear to believe they did. These can manifest as illusions or hallucinations that are based on false assumptions. This could be a general confusion about the passing of time or making up the gaps in their memories, since they've lost their memories regarding what been happening to them in their lives. If this happens Try to gently inform your loved ones that this isn't the case, and then have them go through old photos or a scrapbook of their memories and discover what they recall. However, most of the time it's not worth the effort to engage in a heated debate with the person suffering from dementia, since it could cause them to be irritated further. It could result in anger or conflict that's more difficult for you to handle. If they feel comfortable to share these stories and stories, allow them to continue doing the same.

Walking around and leaving the house Unassisted: It's true that wandering is a typical sort of behaviour in Alzheimer's patients even

12

when it seems innocent or your family member admitting that they're wandering for no reason like going to the bathroom or searching for their medication. It is crucial that , when wandering takes place you have someone watching your loved one at all times. We'll go over this in a subsequent chapter, and will provide safety tips that you need to know and follow.

Chapter 4: Fear Of Violence

It can be difficult to know what to do when a loved one suffering from dementia is acting in a violent manner. Sometimes, their actions can be mentally or physically exhausting and can be extremely difficult for caregivers. The behavior could be related to the person's personality prior to the time they began developing dementia, but it can occur in any person regardless of their prior personality nature. It can be physical or verbal behaviors, and can include a mixture of shouting, screaming or making threats or hitting, biting or pushing and pushing.

Most often, this physical aggression will be triggered by the patient's discontent. They might not understand their needs, be able to meet their desires or speak clearly enough to communicate what they want with you, as the caregiver. There could be a myriad of reasons for this violence that could be the cause, including:

* Side effects of medications and dosage adjustments: This could cause a person to feel sleepy and confused and may even hinder their already low communication skills

14

Overwhelming surroundings: Perhaps they feel that the space they are in is not a suitable environment for their preferences. It could be loud or bright or loud and busy. It could be that it's monotonous and quiet. The stillness is what makes them nervous.

* Vision or hearing loss in the absence of functioning senses can make anyone feel lost and overwhelmed and lost, but it is even more difficult for people with dementia who are having a hard time relying on their mental faculties.

"Hallucinations": Such imaginings can be scary for the person you love dearly and can cause them to believe that what they witnessed is actually happening. If you or a family member is hesitant to doubt the authenticity of these hallucinations the delusions, your loved one could become more assertive when challenged.

* Feeling pain or discomfort You may notice that your loved ones are experiencing an issue with their body that they can't describe. Make sure that they go to regular appointments and undergo regular physical examinations to make sure the absence of physical discomfort.

* Loss of agency The loss of the ability to take care of you and take your own choices could be a snare and your loved ones might be feeling depressed or angry about what they can't accomplish.

If you experience episodes of aggression it is important to know how to deal with it for your own safety and that of the person you love. Before reacting to the situation, take a deep breath and give the person space. Be calm as you don't want to display your anger or frustration, which could make the situation more difficult and aggravate the situation. Avoid expressing any emotion of anxiety or fear as this can cause the individual's anger to grow. If you feel you're in danger you must quit the situation and contact to seek assistance. Make sure you're secure as your safety is vitally crucial.

Give the person enough the space. Avoid initiating physical contact with the person might find it intimidating. One tip is to keep your position and your body language the same to that of the person you are talking with. If they're seated then you should be too. Simulate their body language to ensure that they feel comfortable and doesn't look like an enemy. Maintaining eye contact is a great option.

Be sure to calm the person, and also take note of their emotions. If they're upset discuss why they are feeling that way. If they are nervous, remind them that they're safe and that this is their place. Remember that they are not planning to hurt you However, they must have a reason for communicating with you, even if the message comes out as an angry outburst. Try distracting the person by engaging them in a task that will help them relax.

After the incident is over, remember not to punish the individual for their actions or blame them for it. In the majority of cases their judgement has diminished and they don't know what they did or comprehend the reason why it was risky. Be as positive as you can and continue to maintain the same attitude and routine toward them. Concentrate on the person, and the way they feel and whether they've been able to adjust to their normal.

If you're being the primary caregiver for your loved one, it may be beneficial to speak with someone about how you're feeling. This could be relatives such as a counselor, an advocate, even the general practitioner. If you're not able to talk about the emotions you are experiencing, it could be difficult for you to concentrate and put aside the negative feelings in order to look after the person you love dearly. Make sure that you take time to unwind and enjoy self-care. This means taking a break from work and time spent with your family and friends. family members to make you feel at relaxed.

A counselor or doctor can assist you in identifying the best ways of controlling aggressive behavior of your child. It can also help you identify the signs of trouble. Recognizing the problem is essential so, take time to consider the reasons that could trigger this response for your loved one with dementia. Perhaps it is something related to their lifestyle? Are they experiencing pain or experiencing discomfort? Are they experiencing discomfort due to their environment of socialization or because they're not receiving enough social interaction? What was the date and when did this issue began? Are there any other individuals involved? Find any patterns you observed in the behavior. It is possible to keep a diary, or writing down any information regarding when the behavior is beginning can help you identify patterns. Determine how the person reacts, and attempt to create a plan. If necessary consult with your patient's physician or counselor involved , if believe the situation hasn't been resolved.

Chapter 5: Working With Memory

There is a general agreement with health professionals that stimulating the mind can help slow the decline of Alzheimer's disease and improve memory recall. Numerous studies have shown that people who receive regular brain stimulation could be able communicate and interact more effectively than they did previously and this increased their quality of life overall. The future of this depends on the level that your dear one's is in. If they're in moderate or mild stages, short-term improvement might be possible to stop further decline in cognitive capacity. If the disease has progressed do not feel guilty even if your activities aren't aiding them or you're not experiencing any improvement.

The best benefit of stimulating the brain is that it can be carried out in a group or on an individual basis. If you have a loved one in an inpatient or in a residential facility, the staff probably have put together activities that will keep residents and physically active. However, if your loved one is living in your home as their primary caregiver You can meet their specific needs and suggest activities that match their interests and ability. This personal connection can be extremely beneficial as you make the time to spend together with the person you love dearly.

There are numerous things you can do for your beloved ones mentally active.

Creative Activities include painting, arts and craft projects knit and embroidery, playing instruments or singing.

* These games are a fantastic way to strengthen your child's creativity like the time they played instruments or crochet. It may be difficult to remember these skills , so be patient and help them along by encouraging them when they've forgotten a step. Attending a class at your local community center is a great opportunity to spend time with your friends and also encourage their artistic aspect.

Thinking Activities: Reading puzzles, board games, puzzles Crossword puzzles, Scrabble maze puzzles.

These types of games can be great for encouraging brain activity as well as "exercise" the mind. They could be solo activities that you offer your loved ones while you are working on another project or something you both can do with each other. Aid them whenever they have a problem however, always be supportive for them even if they're dissatisfied that they can't accomplish it on their own.

Physical Activity such as walking and dancing, working out as well as yoga, stretching.

Participating in physical activities is an excellent method to increase exercise levels and keep track of the flexibility and endurance. Naturally, such kinds of activities are prone to being hampered by physical and age-related conditions However, even an easy stroll along the street or taking an elderly yoga class could allow your loved one to remain alert and focused. Exercise can have many benefits, such as boosting your energy as well as ensuring you get an improved night's rest as well as improving the mood of your. Naturally, you do not want to leave your loved ones alone wandering around in case they suffer from significant dementia or have issues with walking. Make sure you accompany them and ensure that they're always monitored when they're attending classes. It is important that the instructor or front desk employee is aware that your loved ones should be kept inside and that you can contact them if they are agitated or seeking to leave.

Social Activities: Senior center activities, classes at the community center socializing with friends and relatives.

* Depending on how advanced the dementia of your loved one is and how well they are able to function in social settings may differ. If the condition is still moderate, they might be at ease in social settings and conversing with others for longer periods of time. If the dementia has advanced it is possible that they forget who the other members of that group is, or they may feel unsafe and become angry. It is your responsibility as a caregiver, to understand the level of their experience and ensure they are never scared or uneasy in a group environment. If they need to, you may take them to classes at the local senior center or community center, to ensure that you're nearby should they become upset or forget where they're. Spending time with friends and family can be a good way to relax people However, ensure that your visits are controlled and not long. Don't cause your loved one to feel they need to play for an extended period of time,

or let something come up which makes them feel angry or upset.

The chores are Setting the table setting on pet food for the day, folding laundry, washing up, washing dishes.

* If your loved one lives with you but doesn't have to do household chores, having them engaged is a good way to let them feel competent. It could be that is as easy as getting the food ready for the evening, or helping wash dishes after dinner. Repeating this practice can help them feel more involved and accountable and decrease their feelings of being in a state of desperation. Always be available to help.

Daily Life Activities include brushing your teeth, eating, dressing and taking a shower or bath.

* It's an excellent idea to review the steps with your child to make sure they're able to perform them correctly. Sometimes , they'll walk out of the bathroom without cleaning their teeth, or feel overwhelmed after taking shower. Be sure to help them along and encourage them, but don't let them feel that they're failing because they've forgotten certain steps.

Reminiscence Therapy involves looking through photos, sharing tales from your past reading old letters, making scrapbooks, and keeping a family tradition alive with specific meals or activities.

* These kinds of activities can help your loved ones improve their memory recall. They don't need to be able to recall particular details however it's a fantastic opportunity to go through their memories and discover the things they can recall without putting pressure on them to remember everything. Research has shown that these kinds of activities have the potential to significantly improve memory recall for people suffering from dementia. However, you must be certain that it's done in a natural way and is designed to be an enjoyable activity rather than being evaluated.

Chapter 6: Speech And Communication Issues

If you're not educated or have trained in communication and speech It can be extremely difficult to talk to people with dementia. After interacting with healthy individuals who are able to clearly convey their ideas, it may be a challenge to be flexible and adapt your manner when talking to someone who is suffering from dementia. However, the more patient you are in your interactions, the better your bond with your loved one be, and it will hopefully bring less stress while you take care of the person.

Here are some helpful tips to help you plan an effective and positive conversation with the person who has dementia.

Be sure that there aren't any distractions. Dementia sufferers can get distracted by the smallest things, like when the television is on, or there's a loud noise from the corners in the space. If you wish to talk to the person , and make sure you're listening make sure you are not distracted by possible noise. Make sure you are in a quieter area when you have to. Attract the attention of the person by saying their name gently and informing them of that you're who you say you're. If they're seated it's also a good idea reach their level of vision and keep eye contact.

Be positive and cheerful. Keep in mind that body language is crucial when talking to someone and you don't know when that your loved one's personality is showing signs of deterioration even in the case of dementia. This is why it's crucial to establish a positive vibe for your loved ones and to maintain a positive attitude and a relaxed body communication. Your facial expressions and voice can be a powerful way to communicate with people, so it is important to remain calm and show respect and affection. Unnecessarily harsh or loud could make someone feel uncomfortable and afraid of you.

Be concise and clear. You should speak slowly and with confident tone. Also, employ simple sentences and words. structures. The more precise and clear you are, the much easier for your audience to follow your instructions. If they aren't able to show that they've grasped the concept initially, think about repeating your message or the question, but make sure that you don't convey anger or discontent in your voice. If someone still does not understand, try rephrasing your inquiry in another manner.

Simple questions can be answered with an "yes" either "no" response. It is best to limit ones questions limited to one question at each time, and make sure you have clear yes or no responses to prevent confusion. Inquiring questions that open up to interpretation can be frustrating for those who ask them if they're not able to formulate a response or remember the question. It is better to state the alternatives you're offering to allow the person to make an informed decision. For example, you could inquire, "Do you want to have a salad with lunch, or a sandwich with grilled cheese?" These two options are laid out clear, and the person who listens hears them so that they can say the option they would prefer. If you ask a question that is open-ended such as, "What would you like to eat for lunch?" the sheer number of options might confuse them.

Be patient and guide them through the tasks by guiding them through a series of steps. This will assist your loved one to make the tasks easier, even the most basic things such as dressing for the day. Remind them gently of the steps like

"Pick out the top you're planning for today's outfit," followed by, "Don't forget to put on your socks when you put on the shoes you're wearing." These simple tips will aid them along the way and will not make them feel embarrassed if they did not follow the steps.

If your loved one is getting annoyed, take them away and redirect their attention. If your loved one is in a state of mind or their level of discomfort in what you're speaking with them or about, they might be angry or frustrated. This is when you must switch topics, or move them to another space to keep them from getting distracted. You could suggest some exercise or purchasing food in the kitchen. Make sure to let them know that you are aware of what they are feeling. For instance, you could say, "I didn't mean to make a comment that could make you feel angry. Let's take a stroll instead." If you are able to acknowledge their emotions, it may assist them in overcoming it and move on towards a new goal.

Be affectionate. Dementia sufferers often feel uneasy about their own situation and that of those around them. They can be confused by events that never occurred and believe that the incidents actually took place. The most effective way you can interact with someone suffering from dementia is to show them love. Keep your eyes on the person's feelings and respond with a calm tone and assurance. Sometimes, physical affection can to calm them down whether it's giving them a hug or holding hands that reminds you of your bond in the way you love about you. The ability to laugh could assist, but make sure your not going to laugh at individual's fault or making jokes about them.

Chapter 7: Home Hazards

The person you love dearly can remain at peace in your home for as long as you're aware of potential hazards and have taken appropriate precautions to protect yourself. Because of the impaired judgement and confusion it is essential that people with dementia are shielded from dangers in the house. Don't leave the door open for an accident to occur which could be a serious act of neglect by you in the event that you've not dealt with the weaknesses within your home.

These are security suggestions to ensure that you have put in place a secure living space for your loved one suffering from Alzheimer's or dementia.

Be sure to assess each room inside your home, as well as the outside. Someone with dementia might wander about the house and wander around areas they're not allowed to even when you've set boundaries for them. Be attentive to all areas , including garages, basements, or areas outside and determine whether anything requires special considerations. Be aware of the areas in which you store medicines and cleaning supplies, or tools, or any other chemicals which must be secured.

Be aware of security hazards that you encounter in your kitchen. If it's knives or the stove, or microwave, make sure to list the hazards within the kitchen. It is possible that you will need to take particular steps to address each risk in a different manner. For instance, ensure you have a safe lock on your drawers to ensure your medicine or knife cabinet is secured. Install a gas shut-off valve , or an electrical breaker next to the stove and ensure that it is shut off after each use and so that the person suffering from dementia is unable to switch on the stove. You could also lock it with child knobs. Make sure that there isn't any cooking seasonings such as sugar or salt lying at the tables in glass containers that might break. This is usually the most hazardous area in the home, and you must make sure you have a thorough inspection.

Make sure that all of your security devices are functioning properly. You should ensure that you have carbon monoxide detectors set up at home in good condition. Make sure you have a fire extinguisher on hand in case you have room.

Most of us don't consider these devices as a necessity, but their presence can save lives! It's only possible only if they're functioning and functioning properly, so make sure you make sure that the batteries are in good condition!

Make sure that the areas you need to access are well-lit. As we've mentioned the elderly are prone to wander around, which is why it's crucial that those areas of your home are lit. This includes entryways, doors as well as stairways and spaces between rooms. Put extra lighting or brighter lighting in areas that require them to prevent falls from occurring. Make sure you remove any obstacles to tripping that could cause accidents. It is important for every route that your loved ones be taking to go to the bathroom or any other part of the house to be clear of obstructions and well-lit.

The bathroom should be safe from injuries. It's a place that is prone to slips and falls in the event that it's not safe for the use of your loved one. Install a walk-in shower in place of a tub with a high edge to allow the person with dementia to get into and out of the tub and out, and also install grab bars to allow them to safely get in and out. Be aware of tiles that slip on the floor, and consider adding textured stickers or water-proofed stickers in place of rugs that slide.

Take away and disable all firearms and other weapons from your house. If you own a gun within your home, it is essential to secure it and secured in all times. The presence of a firearm within the home of someone with dementia could result in many tragic scenarios in the event that they stumble upon it. They may mistakenly view another person in the family as intrusion or turn it off themselves. It is vital to ensure that guns are disabled or completely removed from the area.

Make sure all chemicals are stored securely. Cleaning ammonia, cleaning supplies and washing detergent "pads," and bleach could all be hazardous when a person with dementia comes across these items. Make sure that all these items are placed in hard to reach places or locked shelves so that your loved one is unable to access the items. There could also be hazardous substances in your garage , such as paint spray or thinner. It is important to ensure these are kept away from reach.

Check for extreme temperatures of food and water. People with dementia could not remember to wait until their bath is cool or their meal is cold enough to consume. It is possible to install an thermometer inside your bathtub or purchase shower controls that are auto-adjusted to make sure they don't to burn themselves from the hot water that is scalding.

Keep an emergency contact list. Make sure you have an easily accessible list of emergency numbers and addresses for your loved ones and doctors, as well as the local fire department and police hospitals, as well as poison control centers. Make sure everyone in the home is aware of this list along with the other caregivers who could be looking after your loved one while you are away. Whatever you do to prepared to avoid emergencies you should always be aware of who to contact if there's one.

Chapter 8: Nutrition And Nutrition For Dementia

The mealtimes can be a struggle when you have a loved one who suffers from dementia. As dementia worsens they might not remember to eat, struggle using the kitchen, or have outrages about the food they're served as well as the food they're offered. Even with these challenges every doctor will tell you that healthy nutrition is essential for keeping your loved one fit and healthy. A poor diet can cause health problems like problems with behavior, diabetes or lead to weight loss. It's vital to remain well as a caregiver, too! You're carrying the burden to care for someone you love so you'll require your energy and take care of yourself as well.

You should be able to eat a balanced diet, with various food items. That means fresh vegetables and fruits Whole grains, high-protein, lean meats, and dairy products with low fat. Always ensure that you follow the diet plan that your physician or nutritionist suggests. They will advise you to avoid the consumption of foods that have high cholesterol levels and high levels of saturated fat. A high saturated fat intake can increase the risk of developing cardiovascular disease. Also, avoid refined sugars since they are extremely harmful for those with diabetes. Instead, look for healthier sweet choices like fresh, mature fruit, honey or agave nectar to use as toppings on oatmeal or yogurt. If someone you love has problems with blood pressure You should also be careful not to use too much salt. This could cause hypertension. Instead, opt for natural spices to season your food.

It is also essential that your loved ones stay hydrated and drinks lots of fluids. In many cases, when there is a loss of memory and signs of dementia, sufferers tend to not drink enough fluids and neglect to drink enough water. Dehydration can trigger various other problems, including breathing and heart rate rapidity in a trance, lethargy and faintness being dizzy and experiencing urinary issues. Be sure to give your loved ones enough drinking water all day long, refilling their water bottle and keeping track of their consumption. It is also important to provide meals that are high in liquids like milkshakes, soups healthy smoothies, fresh fruit.

As the disease develops, people tend to lose appetite and weight loss could be an issue to be concerned about. In this instance it is possible that the doctor will suggest adding bar or protein shakes which can provide additional calories. Be aware that the reverse is also possible, in which people may not remember what the food they had! In this case it is best not to continue to remind them that you ate before when they are unable to recall. Instead, serve a variety of smaller meals in a short period of time like cereal or toast, followed by toast or a slice or an assortment of fresh fruit. Make sure you have healthy snacks available when they complain that they're hungry, even if they've only ate. So, at least they're eating something nutritious!

It is also crucial to recognize the causes of a poor appetite that could be affecting the dementia sufferer. It can happen when the person you love dearly doesn't recognize a new food , or is unable to test it. It can also be painful to eat in the event of dental or denture-related issues Make certain that you visit your dentist on a regular basis. As the disease progresses, people's perception of taste and smell tend to decrease, and they might feel the food they eat has gone bland and may not be able to eat. Changes in medications or dosages can affect appetite. If you notice a drastic decrease in appetite, it's crucial that to speak with your physician to determine what you can do.

In the midst of all the difficulties that may arise, eating time can be a struggle. To make eating simpler, here are a few ideas you can use.

Beware of distractions. As we've already mentioned, one of the signs of dementia could be difficulties focussing on a job. This is why you should try to make your mealtimes as relaxing as you can without distractions from outside or with the TV on. Make sure that your space is peaceful, and stay clear of any distractions like work or other activities that may distract your loved ones from enjoying the dinner.

Make sure to check the temperature of your food prior to serving. People with dementia often have trouble being able to determine the temperature of something. This can lead to them burning by touching the hot plates or drink a boiling coffee or soup. As the person who is responsible for their care, make certain that you test the

39

temperature of food and drinks prior to serving. If you serve them hot even if you instruct the child to wait for a few minutes before it cools down, they might not wait long enough, which could lead to burns or an injury.

Encourage independence in eating. Be aware of what your child's capabilities are. If they are able to eat using spoon and fork and fork, encourage them to consume what they want do on their own. If they can't make use of utensils or utensils at all, serve them food items, so that they can be able to eat for themselves. Do not stress about cleanliness, let them eat as many as they want on their own. Make sure that the food you prepare isn't too difficult to swallow or create a choke danger.

Place the food in a dish that allows food to be clearly distinguished from the dish. Many times, changes in visual and spatial capabilities can cause people with dementia to recognize their food items on the plate. Avoid using dishes with patterns as they make it difficult to view your food in a clear way. It is helpful to use simple white bowls and dishes so that your loved ones are able to clearly observe the food's color as well as texture and size.

Accept changes to your food preferences. Be aware that dementia could cause someone to change their minds about certain food items. It is possible that your loved one may suddenly be able to enjoy foods they've never enjoyed previously, or turn off foods they've always loved. Be sure to keep an optimistic mood and remain open to changes!

Enjoy meals as a family, if you are able to. Make mealtimes as pleasurable and comfortable as you can so that everyone feels at ease with each other. So everyone is looking eagerly to being together, and enjoying a tasty and nutritious food. This makes it a moment that your loved ones enjoys instead of looking forward to.

Give them time to consume food. One of the last things you'd like to do is to rush the individual to eat, which can make the mealtime a more stressful experience. Consider that your patient with dementia could have a longer time eating. Their mind may be distracted, or they might be distracted by their thoughts, and it could take them more the time needed to sample and chew each bite. It can take up to at least an hour for them to finish their meal and be satisfied with what they consumed. Be patient and ensure that you have enough time to prepare your dinner.

Chapter 9: Daily Exercises

Similar to food and dietary needs You should make sure that you've spoken with the doctor for your loved one about physical activity. There might be medical concerns specific to individual physical issues, but most doctors recommend gentle exercises that can increase flexibility and blood circulation, as well as strength, and the quality of sleep. It's a fantastic mood boost and can boost your energy too! The more active and limber your loved ones are in their later years and the longer they are able to stay active for longer and enjoy an active, better living quality.

It can be difficult at first to get your loved one to engage in exercise, particularly in the past when they've been hesitant. To counter this, make it as a pastime instead of a chore for example, a dance event or a yoga class with soothing music. It could be helpful to train them along with them. This will increase their confidence even if they don't remember the steps, and they will be able to emulate your moves. Additionally, isn't it more enjoyable to exercise with a partner?

It doesn't need to be a difficult workout , or even the physical effort of leaving your home. It's just about finding the time and making some effort. For those who are new to the sport who are just starting out, starting with 10 to 15 minutes couple of times per week is ideal. After that, perhaps scheduling 20-25-minute block sessions every day. Don't overdo it in the beginning as it could lead to injury.

There are many benefits to exercising, as we've mentioned earlier and you could be able to see improvements in your loved ones' overall well-being. This includes things such as:

* slowing down mental decline

* lessening the chance of depression

Improved heart health

* aiding them in sleeping faster and improving their sleep quality

* reduce the symptoms of constipation, diarrhea and indigestion.

* increasing balance and flexibility

* lessening stress and improving mood

* lessening episodes of agitation or wandering caused by mood fluctuations

Safety is foremost and that's the reason you must ensure that you consult your doctor prior to making any changes to your loved one's routine. Make sure that you're in the room and watching the level of effort, ensuring you can ensure that it's a safe pace. Be sure that they are hydrated and taking breaks as needed. If you experience any signs that you are weak, dizzy or pain you should stop right away and take a take a break.

What simple exercises that can be completed by those who suffer from dementia? Here are some suggestions you could try.

* Walking: It's an exercise that is simple and is often not thought of as an exercise! A walk around the backyard, around the house or even down the block is an ideal way to get breath, move your legs and release some energy. If you know someone who isn't keen on exercise be sure to disguise it in ways that get the person involved, like going for a dog stroll or walking along the street to visit a friend's home.

* Work on balance: Maintain your balance when standing up by holding the objects you require to support yourself, then make an effort to keep your balance against the wall while in sitting

posture. This exercise will improve your the balance and posture of your body in the course of time.

Stretching simply stretching your body will help relieve stiff muscles and alleviate joint pain. It is possible to do it with assistance or on its own. It is not uncommon to find a massage is a fantastic option to soothe sore muscles as well!

* Tai Chi, Yoga Pilates and Tai Chi They tend to be less intense and are more stretching, which is perfect for seniors. Try following a workout on the internet or attending classes in your local fitness center. You can modify them according to the physical demands of your loved ones.

* House chores: They can be an excellent opportunity to "sneak" into exercising for your loved ones without them even knowing. They will be involved in household chores and competent to do their part. Things like dusting the home, light vacuuming and washing dishes require motor skills.

* Gardening If you know someone who is a gardener and is a lover of gardening this is an ideal idea for them to get engaged in. It's exercise that doesn't feel like being a burden! The act of

pulling weeds, shoveling or raking are an excellent workout. Plus, you'll be able to watch your flower garden and vegetable garden increase in size as well!

* Exercises in the water: These are considered to be excellent for older people, since there's no strain on joints when you're swimming. It is a fantastic method to ease the pain of arthritis as well as the pressure on joints. It also functions as a type of resistance, which means you can do strength training without the need for weights! The local senior center or gym is likely to offer a range of classes in water aerobics for older adults.

* Dancing: It can be a great activity for socializing which also provides physical exercise. If you know someone who enjoys dancing or is a fan of a particular kind of dance like dance, salsa, and waltz this could be an excellent way to get them back on their feet and back on their feet! You can set the music at home and host the dance of your dreams or check the elderly center, or retirement facility offers dance classes or events for your loved ones to go to.

Chapter 10: Wandering Issues

The elderly are more likely to wander around aimlessly. It could be a adverse effects of certain medications, or boredom in their surroundings, or they may claim that they are "looking at some thing" or someone, but are uncertain of where that individual or thing is. They might say they're hungry thirsty, hungry, or simply require a bathroom. Such behavior could cause anxiety for caregivers and can be frightening particularly if you live living in a place that has stairs or has hazards just around the corner. It's crucial to spend the time to identify any reasons for wandering, and take the necessary measures to limit any danger.

Here are some ideas that can aid you in identifying someone you love who is inclined to wander.

* Attach child-safe plastic covers for doors or drawers that you don't want the child to get into such as the medicine drawer, as well as cutlery as well as knife drawers.

Make sure that the person is exercising regularly. It can help people feel less agitated and that they've had the time to wander around the house or outside that day and that they don't have to wander around to satisfy curiosity.

Install a home security or a monitoring system that will monitor the person, particularly if you're away from home or you don't have anyone in the house to supervise them. If the system is equipped with speakers, so that you can speak to the person you are monitoring and provide them with directions, it's an excellent way to soothe the person if they appear to be wandering about the home.

Consider an GPS device that can be used to determine the location of a person if they leave. It can be added to a watches or put on a necklace to ensure that you are able to find the person if they leave.

You can use barriers such as curtains or a visible STOP sign to remind your loved ones that they must not continue past this threshold.

Make sure that your loved ones are wearing an identification bracelet. In the event that they go off and fail to remember their name or provide specific information, their name as well as address will be recognized by others. Take a photo of your loved one to use for identification reasons.

• Inform your neighbors of the issues with wandering and make certain they are aware of the need to contact you in the event that they see someone in the yard or outside the area of the house.

Consider installing locks which require new key. It is best to put them either high or low on the door, as people with dementia tend to glance at their eyes. It is important to distribute keys to the other family members so that you can account for possible fire hazards or security concerns. Don't make life difficult for the your household members!

Chapter 11: Handling Mood Changes

As a caregiver for people with dementia and their families, it's important to be aware of any mood changes that may happen. This could be due to medications side effects, anger over their decline in cognitive capabilities or simply being in a bad mood the mood swings could occur suddenly. They can include moods such as:

* Apathy
* depression
* Angry
* anger
* Affliction
* nervousness
* Fear or anxiety
* Overreaction
* Hyperstimulation
* Sadness

These mood swings can make it difficult to determine what to do with your beloved one. It is crucial to be aware of what you can do and don't appear dissatisfied or shocked by the changes in their mood. This could cause them to behave further. Remember that it's not your responsibility. The dementia is taking over their senses, often causing their emotions erratic.

Here are some helpful tips we can give you on how to handle mood swings to make it a more pleasant experience for you and the loved ones who suffers from dementia.

Be sure to take complaints of pain seriously. If someone is claiming they're hurting or experiencing trouble, try not to dismiss it even if they tend to tell false or untrue statements or even make up false claims. Do not want the perception to be one of injured and that it was not noticed. Make sure you inquire about their feelings. Are they exhausted? Hungry? Sleepy? Thirsty? What's the source of pain? Take note of how they feel and check for physical bruises or marks in their physique.

Be sure that the person is engaged in sufficient activities. Sometimes, mood swings may result from fatigue or boredom. Be sure that your loved one has plenty of activities to engage in throughout the day, and has enough time for rest and sleep too. Are they exercising enough? Do they prefer early morning or late evening walk? Do they prefer being outside or inside? Are they engaged enough in mind-training activities such as playing games or reading to keep them amused? You should ensure that your routine includes enough things to keep their attention and allow them the time to unwind and relax. It is important to establish a routine they're happy with and do not make any abrupt changes that could result in discontent.

Assist them in completing those tasks that cause them to be frustrated. When someone cannot recall how to complete a task and is frustrated, they can get angry and suffer an emotional swing. If you notice something similar to this is happening or you realize that they're feeling anxious about a specific job, such as helping to with the setting of up the tables or running their hair through, make sure you take the time to finish the task together with them. This will help refresh their memory and increase their confidence.

Make sure you create a peaceful and tranquil setting. Even if you lead an active home life that involves lots of people from and away, make sure that the person who has dementia is always comfortable in the home. is a comfortable and safe area. This could include setting something such as "quiet time" to ensure that they are at peace, or even directing teens or children to play in a different area of the home if the noise level is bothering the person you love dearly. Unexpected noises or interruptions to their

54

routines could trigger mood swings in your loved one, so make sure to set schedules that will put them at ease and aren't likely to frighten them.

Offer a distraction. This could be an attempt to avoid the situation however sometimes switching the topic and providing an opportunity to distract yourself can help you avoid a major meltdown or emotional situation. Consider if they would like drinks or snacks or would like to go for an excursion around the house or out. Perhaps you could mention that you have an appointment to complete or a project to complete , and they'll be able to help. Sometimes, simply taking their minds away from the issue can bring them back to their happy mood.

Be sure to keep your goodbyes short. Most of the time, if you leave your home for an outing or need be able to leave a loved one who has dementia for a couple of hours, it can result in a lot of stress in the person. There is a chance that those who are following them that they feel a shift in their mood and can be difficult to cope with for a few days afterwards. To avoid this type of behavior change ensure that your goodbyes are short so that you don't upset them. Do not tell someone that you'll be leaving frequently, as they may be stressed out more. Be natural, and then tell them that you'll be leaving and will be back within a couple of hours. This will make it easier for them to understand that they're not focusing on your departure.

When in doubt, get help. If you suspect that your loved one is experiencing trouble with their moods and you're not seeing any positive changes, don't hesitate seeking help from your counselor of senior or their general practitioner. They might have some answers for you on the subject of their mood fluctuations or determine whether the cause is with their medications or dosage. They could be able suggest activities to try and engage in, or treatments that have demonstrated improvement. It's fine to seek assistance!

Chapter 12: Additional Helpful Tips

caring for someone suffering from dementia can be challenging as well as an initial process of learning. Don't be discouraged if find it difficult to do it, as it can be! This book will give you useful tips and suggestions on how to manage certain situationsto ease the stress you feel and create an easier and more relaxing setting for you and your loved ones suffering from dementia.

Here are some additional tips that caregivers from all walks of life have shared with you to assist in your way.

The argument may result in you being both annoyed. It is frustrating when your loved one says things that aren't true or is telling false stories or reliving memories repeatedly. However, you must keep in mind that it's not their fault; it's the disease which is altering their minds. They believe in the things they say, because that's the message their brains are telling them. It is tempting to debate and make corrections but you can't overcome a disagreement when someone's logic and judgment is changed. This could result frustrated for both you and trigger emotional turmoil in the person you love. Remember to let some fights go.

Cognitive exercises don't waste time. It's not too late to test to enhance your loved one's cognitive abilities. It can be difficult to believe that they're "too distantly away," but remind yourself that you're spending time with your loved one, and creating memories with your beloved one. Keep working on activities like puzzles, painting crafting, or whatever else your loved one would enjoy. They are all beneficial for those suffering from dementia.

Make a list of what is important to you, and then learn to let go of the rest. It is a fact that people who suffer from dementia aren't going to be able do everything flawlessly. You must learn what is important to them as their caretaker. Perhaps you would prefer that you maintain their hygiene. Maybe it's more important for you to have them in the kitchen with the family. Make sure your loved one is safe and keep them in your thoughts to assist them in completing the tasks that are important to you. Relax in the event that exercises or artistic pursuits have been put on the schedule for a couple of days.

Sometimes, all they require. If you see an increase in mood or someone you love becomes stressed or combative, the best thing you could offer them is some time to relax. Be sure you are secure if they enter their bedroom or in any room they're in. However, you should you should leave the area for 10-15 minutes so that each of you can relax and reflect on the situation. It could be that when you return to investigate a different approach the person is happier and are more open to what you have to say.

Keep yourself informed about the medication your loved person is taking. The majority of medications are prescribed to treat symptoms of dementia. However, your loved one might be suffering from other conditions other than dementia that require medication, for example, high blood pressure, diabetes or high blood pressure, for instance. One of the most important ways to help is to keep track of the dosage they are taking as, more often than not you're the one providing it. It is also essential to be aware of how specific medications affect your brain and the potential adverse consequences. So, you'll be able to determine if a new behaviors are related to medications or if it is something that should be reported to your doctor. It is also crucial to have your doctor review any changes that could be made to your loved one's medications or supplements, diet and workout routines. It's better to inquire more questions than not enough!

Be prepared for the difficult conversations you have to. The subjects of a will, living will as well as power of attorney can be challenging to discuss with someone you love since they are only able to bring up our mortality. But discussing these options and completing the paperwork prior to the onset of a medical emergency is essential, to ensure that things can be resolved quickly. You'll want to ensure that your loved one is in a positive mindset to respond to these questions and are content with the responses. The majority of loved ones will experience an increased sense of calm when they know that they will be honored in their wishes.

Be sure to take care of yourself! Caring for others can be a stressful and exhausting job, particularly in the case of being on your own or with other responsibilities. You should have a network that can offer help when you're overwhelmed and also someone that you can talk to about the difficulties that you're facing. Alongside other family members or acquaintances you should try to join an organization that supports caregivers or an older group in your neighborhood center or retirement facility. Take time breaks during the course of your day even if it's only one hour of your time to relax and unwind when your loved one takes nap. Health is vital as well!

Chapter 13: What's Alzheimer's Disease?

It is one of the prevalent kind of degenerative brain disease that is most commonly affecting the older people (over 65 being the highest typical age for it to manifest). Alzheimer's is known for its memory loss, impairment of short-term memory, difficulties in comprehending language or speaking and problem-solving, disorientation mood swings, as well as behavior issues. The condition usually begins slow and gradually gets worse and can affect the ability to do everyday tasks and care for themselves until they are unable to swallow or breathe on their own without assistance. The most prevalent reason for dementia. Around 60 to 80 percent of cases of dementia result from Alzheimer's disease however, it is not uncommon for someone to have more than one form of. Women are significantly more likely to develop the disease . 65 percent of patients with the condition are females with reasons that are only speculated on.

It is difficult to know for certain about the illness and there isn't an universally accepted cure or any preventative treatment. Numerous studies show various results and even homeopaths, doctors and health professionals promote contradictory assertions.

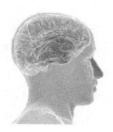

While some preventative measures have been proven to be effective but no solution has proved to be successful in all instances. One of the challenges in finding the cure is that there isn't a method to detect Alzheimer's disease in living people, and so sometimes it's difficult to tell that a person is suffering from Alzheimer's until symptoms become evident. One way to be able to tell that for sure is through post-mortem exams, which show two types of abnormalities that are linked with the disease: neurofibrillary Tangles and plaques of beta-amyloid. Tangles are a mass of altered proteins in brain cells, which block essential chemicals and nutrients from being transferred from one area of the cell and plaques are proteins that form between nerve cells, instead of being flushed away. Plaques block chemical flow and communication between neurons, and tangles block signals and chemicals from passing through the cell. This results in cells not being able to get the proper amount of chemicals and then deteriorating or dying. Tangles and plaques also cause the accumulation of waste proteins as well as harmful chemicals which the brain isn't in a position to flush.

The entire brain shrinks drastically as the illness gets worse. Further research has shown that inflammation at a cellular scale triggered by toxic substances, stress or head injuries and is linked to Alzheimer's Disease contributes to the demise of neurons.

Although there isn't a consensus-based method to reverse the damage done by the illness at the moment, there are a variety of generally accepted preventative methods including non-invasive therapies that incorporate mental exercise good diet, physical fitness, regular sleep and social interaction to stop the progression of the disease, however there is no agreement on their effectiveness in the minds of doctors and scientists.

Research into Alzheimer's disease treatment is among the most heavily funded areas that is making progress at a rapid speed, making it difficult to discern the most recent findings and reliable, and which information is has been dated. The primary part of the brain to develop plaques and tangles is called the hippocampus. The hippocampus is two areas of brain with one on each side which look similar to two seahorses. The hippocampus is accountable for short-term memory, long-term memory, as well as spatial navigation. These are the most common cognitive problems those suffering from Alzheimer's experience. The majority of people with Alzheimer's have smaller hippocampuses when the disease begins. This is different from others who are similar to them - it is believed that certain regions that are part of our brains shrink as a result of inactivity , making it more prone to developing plaques and knots. Although brain shrinkage is thought to be to be common among the elderly however, it is not by any by any means a natural or inevitable aspect of the process of aging.

The condition was first discovered through Alois Alzheimer around 1907 after he observed abnormal protein deposits within the brain of his elderly patient after she had passed from the disease. The protein collection was vastly different from what he'd previously seen, so he declared it as a new disease. Alzheimer's disease was not mentioned frequently in the medical publications and journals until the 1970's , and before that time, it was only discussed as a rare illness. Since then, there's been a sharp rise in deaths due to Alzheimer's disease and other forms of dementia which has led many doctors to ask if the modern environments, stress, modern lifestyles and changes to diet may play a role in the development of the disease. The fact that people live longer than they did 100 years ago could be a factor in why many people are suffering from this condition.

However, this doesn't explain the dramatic rise that we have witnessed in recent years and the findings which predicts a further growth in the coming years. It is crucial to be aware that many people reach an older age with no evidence of loss of memory and there is no evidence of tangles or plaques in post-mortem research, whereas some have tangles and plaques and have a strong cognitive function when they die.

Memory loss among older people, though normal and generally harmless however, it is not a normal process of aging. Rather, it is a result of neural damageand other different forms of dementia. Alzheimer's disease is a devastating form of dementia due to the fact that the decline of the patient is swift. As opposed to other forms of dementia Alzheimer's disease is a disease that affects all areas of neuronal functioning, which includes the automatic bodily functions such as breathing and swallowing.

The ability to communicate and comprehend rapidly and patients require round-the-clock 24/7 care right after the onset illness. It is often referred to as the most costly illness - when you consider the cost of treatment as well as physical treatment as along with the expanding market of drugs, pharmaceuticals and homeopathic treatments nursing homes, and many more.

There's a lot of debate in the research and treatment of Alzheimer's. Homeopathic remedies have been discredited as unsubstantiated or untrue in research, and in the same time, more than 99% of the drugs used during clinical studies have been proven to be ineffective (Forbes; Promising Alzheimer's Treatments fail to impress with new data). It is essential to stay aware of and critical of treatments , and be aware of any adverse side effects and potential complications.

The speed of progression from moderate to extreme varies from person to. As the disease advances functional and cognitive abilities decrease. Individuals require help with everyday activities like bathing, eating, dressing, and going to the bathroom. They also lose their ability to communicate, fail to identify loved ones and then become dependent on their bed. If people have trouble moving they are more susceptible to infection, including the pneumonia (infection of the lung).

Pneumonia caused by Alzheimer's is often a contributor in the deaths of those who suffer from Alzheimer's disease.

Chapter 14: The Early Signs And Symptoms Of Alzheimer's

As opposed to leukaemia and cancer the Alzheimer's disease is one without a biomarker, which means there isn't a scan, blood test, or procedure that can be carried out on a person who is living to determine if they suffer from the disease. Alzheimer's is diagnosed based on the symptoms and behaviors of the patient, once the other causes are eliminated. Post-mortem examination is the only way to determine the specific plaques and tangles that define the condition.

Therefore, Alzheimer's disease is generally diagnosed when symptoms have significantly worsened. Some health experts believe that Alzheimer's starts to progress long before symptoms become apparent. The changes within the brain are thought to begin 20 years prior to the onset of symptoms. One test employs EEG (electrical activities) patterns, and is considered to be an precise, non-invasive method to determine if you have Alzheimer's. It is widely known that patients affected by the disease show more or less intense electrical activity in particular regions of their brain. EEG patterns can be used to detect small changes in these regions which begin to show a noticeable changes in activity as early as 10 years prior to the onset of symptoms. This implies that electrical activity can be used to identify Alzheimer's disease early.

A lot of health professionals, particularly neurologists Dr. Reisa Sperling, advocate for early diagnosis of Alzheimer's disease as people can delay or stop its effects through the right physical and mental activities as well as a balanced diet.

The most prevalent process of developing Alzheimer's disease from the time of diagnosis until death is in a time span of between 3 and 9 years, and is known as"the Alzheimer's continuum. The Alzheimer's continuum usually begins with those over 65, however some individuals - as high as to 5% diagnosed prior to this. The initial stage of Alzheimer's that is not able to be diagnosed officially is known as pre-dementia. It is characterised by small-scale memory loss, which is usually dismissed as normal memory loss or trouble concentrating. Some doctors believe that there is no any kind of memory loss that isn't natural even for the elderly. Any symptoms of memory loss could be an indication of dementia.

The initial signs of Alzheimer's disease that are eligible as clinical signs is memory loss and impairment of cognitive function which interferes with everyday life. The signs and symptoms differ from individual to individual. The ability to learn and remember are often the first areas of cognitive function that suffer however, some individuals may are experiencing difficulties with perception, language coordination, and movement as the initial signs.

The new information can be difficult to remember and learn more seasoned memories, information acquired earlier in the life of the individual and routines are usually less affected in the initial stages of the illness.

A renowned neurologist Dr. Majid Fohuti warns against getting overwhelmed and focusing too much on the onset of symptoms. The public should be aware of the signs and find ways of dealing with these, or adopting lifestyle changes to make up for the issues. Doctor. Fohuti explains that there is a anxiety that surrounds the diagnosis of Alzheimer's and it is crucial to make sure that memory loss is not misinterpreted as a sign of progression to Alzheimer's disease. Here are some signs of Alzheimer's disease, as well as typical instances of loss of memory which do not necessarily signal the presence of Alzheimer's disease.

Memory Loss that can interfere with daily activities

Alzheimer's patients tend to forget new information and may have difficulty remembering simple details. This can include forgetting the same information repeatedly like dates and names for example, or not being able to recall recent events like the food you had for breakfast or how you cleaned your teeth. It is common for people to record things in a different way than they did previously or rely on others to remind them of events. A typical moment of forgetfulness is when you forget the name of a person or an appointment and being able to recall the event later.

Trouble with Tasks that are familiar

The tasks that didn't cause any difficulty prior to becoming difficult for people suffering from

Alzheimer's disease. Things like driving on a familiar route becomes complicated task, or a person losing the ability to play a certain game can indicate the progress of Alzheimer's.

It is common to slip up or make mistakes you aren't sure how to correct yourself like accidentally changing the settings on your phone.

Issues with Problem Solving or planning

Alzheimer's disease impacts people's ability to concentrate and to process a situation or formulate a plan that includes various steps. For instance , some people be unable to follow a recipe for recipe for cooking, arranging their schedules and managing their bills. It is becoming more difficult to use as Alzheimer's disease advances. Some people may have difficulty using a device they're familiar with, for example, microwaves or mobile phones.

A difficult time integrating the new technology or need help to fix the settings of the device are common issues seniors will face.

Problem with Spatial Relationships of Perception

Alzheimer's patients may struggle to comprehend what they see - such as judging distance, distinguishing objects, or recognizing the difference between color and contrast. This is especially dangerous for drivers. Reading can be difficult because it can be difficult to comprehend the alphabet on a page. This kind of vision problem is a result of brain damage and not in the eyes. those who suffer from cataracts or are short or far-sighted as they age don't have the same difficulties.

The changes in Mood and Personality

Memory and understanding problems are often caused by mood changes and personality. The signs can be scary and individuals can be irritable and anxious, as well as confused or fearful. They are prone to becoming angry with relatives and friends at times without any apparent reason. Many patients are unaware of their conditions and are not conscious of their issues and can become frustrated when they feel that people are acting odd in their presence for no reason. When they are forced away from their normal routine individuals with Alzheimer's disease may be irritated and even anger. Being upset when a routine routine is disturbed is normal, as is being angry in the event of fatigue.

Problems with Language

People suffering from Alzheimer's disease may struggle to remember the correct word when writing or speaking. They might lose a popular word or require replacing it by using a different phrase or word. They might have trouble understanding the flow of conversation or taking part in one. Sometimes, they be unable to finish an exchange without being able to remember the words they were trying to say as well as repeating the same sentence repeatedly. Sometimes, you may forget a word you are able to recall later on, however, does not suggest a loss of memory due to Alzheimer's disease.

Unusual dates or places

The difficulty in retaining spatial memory and numbers is a sign the presence of Alzheimer's. People are prone to forgetting the date, time or even struggle to comprehend the time passing by. Some people forget where they came from or even forget the location they're in. The habit of forgetting the date of the week or losing track of duration of time while doing something exciting is a common occurrence, but is different from the norm, and is not a sign of Alzheimer's disease.

Losing Things

Alzheimer's patients are more likely to lose objects and are unable to find them. They are often able to place objects in a particular place and not be in a position to locate items. It can become more frequent and challenging as the condition progresses, and may lead to them accusing other people of taking things. The habit of sloppyly putting things away at times, but being able retrace your steps to locate it, is a normal occurrence for people who are elderly.

Poor Judgement

Alzheimer's sufferers can make quick decisions when the illness affects their judgment. They can suddenly shift their views regarding religion or politics for example or be obsessed with new diets or pay large sums of money to Telemarketers. In the same way, they are less attentive to their well-being and health. Making a poor decision such as a purchase made in haste and then coming to recognize that it was reckless later, is a normal.

Refrain from Social Activities Regularly

When daily tasks become difficult, people suffering from Alzheimer's might begin withdrawing from social gatherings, work or quit activities and hobbies they used to enjoy. They might be annoyed or ashamed of their inability to complete things and not be social due to this. This is very different from having to take a longer nap when you age, or being exhausted or exhausted due to too many obligations.

The moderate phase that the illness is associated by progressive decline that dramatically impacts the patient's ability to manage their health. Patients may lose the capacity to comprehend their condition and limitations. The ability of a person to talk gets affected as he/she experiences difficulties remembering words and frequently is using the wrong word. Memory becomes increasingly shaky and the person is unable to recognize their relatives.

Around 30 percent of patients at this stage experience illusionary symptoms and mistaken identification. Personality and behavior changes can also begin to manifest, with patients becoming angry and crying out in a flash, or getting aggressive or refusing the care. In the later stages of Alzheimer's disease, patients are completely dependent on their caregivers. Patients are unable to speak or communicate at all, although they frequently they can comprehend when asked and show some indications of comprehension. Inability to complete most tasks the patient can become restless and eventually bedridden with a significant reduction in muscle mass. In contrast to other types of dementia, the patient's primary motor abilities are affected by the illness such as breathing and the ability to swallow. The majority of patients die due to an additional illness, such as pressure ulcers or pneumonia.

Chapter 15: The Believed As The Causes Of The Disease

The cognitive difficulties associated with Alzheimer's disease arise from the accumulation in tangles, plaques inside and around neural cells which result in the death of cells. This is all well-known and has been confirmed. What is the cause of these plaques or tangles appear is remains a mystery. research and studies haven't verified any of the theories.

Certain factors that lead to the development of the disease are well-known. Certain genetic mutations can be related to Alzheimer's disease, and in particular those that are early-onset Alzheimer'. There's certainly a major genetic factor that causes the type of Alzheimer's that is late-onset but research suggests that even those who are thought to be at risk of getting Alzheimer's disease don't always develop it. This leads researchers to conclud that genetics is a crucial but not the only factor that plays a role in the development of Alzheimer's disease.

The dramatic rise in Alzheimer's disease in recent years suggests that it's a condition that is a result of modern lifestyles and diet. Numerous studies have shown that the absence of mental stimulation throughout one's life can contribute to the development of Alzheimer's disease. The current sedentary lifestyle and the absence of physical and mental activities have been found as a risk factor for getting dementia. Feeling lonely, depressed or engaging in a passive, mental activity such as watching television for extended periods of time are all contributing to the progression of dementia. Also, lack of sleep and stress during life speed the progression of the condition, because the brain is constantly pushed and fatigued, and due to lack of sleep, the brain doesn't have enough time to replenish and eliminate the toxins.

Sleep deprivation can lead to more difficulty learning, memory loss and an increase in tau protein in the brain The protein is can be found in neurotangles in Alzheimer's disease.

The results of studies show that people from western countries sleep less, and are stressed out more often than they used to. A study has shown that people who experience feelings of being lonely have 1.63 percent more likely suffer from dementia. In the current highly connected and social media-based world, there's plenty of communication, however people are reported to feel less connected from one another.

A repeated head injury could cause Alzheimer's disease, and can also cause severe blows to the head, which can cause disruption to brain functioning. Due to the increasing popularity of sports that involve high-contact and the increasing number of car accidents, it's not a surprising that brain injuries have become now more common in our society today. Boxers, war veterans football players, and those who have been involved in serious accident in their cars are all more likely be diagnosed with dementia.

The rise of metals and toxins in the food and environment is directly connected to the development of Alzheimer's disease. The long-term exposure to aluminium and silicon exposure to toxins in environmental sources, and free radical damage have all been recognized as the main causes of the condition. Particularly, aluminium has been identified as a potential cause as the metal's toxic effects have been detected in neurofibrillary tangles. We don't know whether aluminium bonds to the tangles when they form or if it is the cause however, studies suggest that aluminum could be a major factor in the development of the condition. Aluminium is found in a variety of unlikely locations today, including every aspect from baking flour, to aluminium cookware, antiperspirant, and deodorant. Studies have shown that aluminum is not a factor in food cooked in a pan for example, unless when it comes to high acidic foods.

Dr. David Perlmutter associates the heavy consumption of carbohydrates and grains with the rise in Alzheimer's and degenerative diseases that is supported by numerous other physicians. He says that the blood brain barrier which controls proteins that get into the cerebral cortex, gets damaged due to gluten. Additionally, gluten can affect the absorption of toxic contaminants and harmful proteins within the intestinal tract. In both cases, it affects how proteins enter and circulate throughout your body.

Dr. Joel Wallach presents a convincing argument the Alzheimer's condition is medically caused illness. The research he conducted shows that

Alzheimer's diseases result from mineral deficiencies and the diet that is poor for many people - rich in carbohydrates, but low in minerals, vitamins saturated fats, cholesterol and vitamins. Wallach claims the doctors mislead patients by prescribing a diet low in cholesterol and dispensing statin medications (which reduce cholesterol) to combat Alzheimer's disease. Cholesterol is a crucial nutrients that are essential to health. The doctor Dr. Wallach contests the fact cholesterol is a factor in heart disease. He also stresses the importance of cholesterol for brain functioning.

75 percent of the brain is made up of a protein known as Myelin and is almost 100% cholesterol. He writes that our culture's anxiety about cholesterol is what has led us not to touch eggs or remove the skin from our chickens in order to be healthy, however, this fear of cholesterol is the exact reason responsible for the dramatic increase in Alzheimer's. If someone were to eat the recommended diet and exercise regularly, within six to 10 years, the individual would be extremely lacking in cholesterol.

Chapter 16: Prevention And Treatment For

Alzheimer's

There is no well-known or proven method to prevent or treat Alzheimer's disease, and researchers scientists, doctors, and homeopaths are engaged in a constant battle over which studies are bogus while promoting their respective cures. The condition is a perpetual market for cures and treatments unfortunately, a lot of people profit from selling expensive treatments or huge amounts of money for the purpose of testing new medications. It is always recommended to consult with your doctor before seeking treatment and to be aware of the entire variety of treatments available and their associated costs, as well as the adverse effects, and long-term effects prior to deciding on an appropriate treatment strategy.

Many doctors suggest considering both the benefits stated and negative effects and risks from any therapy. One treatment approach is using B12 supplements or solving crosswords for ten minutes every day could help with the condition without necessarily affecting your the daily routine. But, there are many treatments that are not as safe. For example one study recently found that Targretin is a drug that was hailed by many as a breakthrough drug and was approved for the treatment of Alzheimer's disease, was not in fact a drug that had any effect on the condition but instead caused a variety of negative side consequences (Forbes: "As More Alzheimer's Treatments Failed, Researchers Discover Possibilities in Vitamins and spice"). The research into Alzheimer's disease is difficult with even groups of researchers and scientists aren't immune to mistakes, but in this case , it can cause severe harm to the health of a lot of people.

As of now there are only six medications that were approved by the U.S. Food and Drug Administration to temporarily ease those suffering from Alzheimer's. They can reduce or stop the degeneration of neurons that is typical of Alzheimer'sdisease. The drugs are only able to provide short-term relief through inundating neurons with neurotransmitter substances. The efficacy of the drugs can vary from individual to individual. There are many reasons finding a reliable drug for treating Alzheimer's disease is so challenging. Human brains are extremely delicate and difficult to locate. It is difficult to work on and nerves are unable to regenerate. In addition, few medications can pass through the blood-brain-barrier that regulates which cells or particles, proteins and even proteins are allowed to enter the brain via the bloodstream. As a result, certain types of drugs do not be absorbed to the brain. Clinical trials and drug development are extremely expensive and take for a lengthy period of time , particularly when it comes to Alzheimer's disease, which is an illness that develops slowly.

Additional medications are prescribed to address specific signs of Alzheimer's disease, such as for instance anxiety or psychosis. These drugs can ease certain symptoms but do not have an influence on the progress of the disease the disease itself. Vitamin E provides antioxidant supplement that can be used in large quantities to treat certain instances with Alzheimer's. Vitamin E must be prescribed by a doctor since it may cause side effectsand may interact with other antioxidants as well as medications. Vitamin E in high doses is known to increase the risk of dying in people suffering from heart issues.

Studies have shown that vitamin E helps protect brain cells from damage caused by chemicals. In another study higher levels of vitamin E have shown lasting effects on slowing the development of Alzheimer's disease.

Recent research is focusing on prevention and the development of methods for combating the signs of Alzheimer's instead of resorting treatment options that are invasive or pharmaceutical which could prove to be more harmful than useful. Alzheimer's disease is linked with stress, insufficient sleep, poor nutrition and the lack of physical activity and social isolation. Although preventative measures do not guarantee that they will work but they can reduce the risk of getting the disease. It is more sensible to establish a healthy routine which will slow the deterioration of your mental health so that the illness doesn't impact people at all. The use of preventative measures has been shown to slow the progression of the condition, even for people who are genetically predisposed to it. A groundbreaking research center called Neurexpand has come up with simple tests for memory and brain exercises that combat the degeneration of the brain with the passage of time, proving that physical exercise, particularly in the beginning phases of Alzheimer's disease,, could combat the negative effects of plaques and tangles of Alzheimer's disease by helping the brain develop pathways around obstructions (Prevention.com).

Like as Dr. Miia Kivipelto points out that we are aware the benefits of a healthy, balanced lifestyle. can be beneficial, however, it's hard to define what constitutes a healthy lifestyle. For example, the precise workouts and diets recommended by doctors differ from one doctor to the next although certain elements are recommended by numerous doctors. This article provides an overview of the suggested physical and mental exercises, as well as the nutritional suggestions from homeopaths who are certified and health experts who are respected.

Chapter 17: The Function Of A Well-Balanced

Diet In Preventing And Curing The Disease

In the past decade, groundbreaking research has connected gut bacteria and nutrition to behavior and learning and have opened a new avenue of study into the interrelations of various organs in the body. In essence, what you consume affects the way you think. Food and nutrition are essential for the health of your brain. Nutritional health is believed to play a greater impact than genetic predisposition to the disease, and may delay the time it takes to develop in those with a high risk. Contrary to genetic predisposition the way you eat is something you control.

One of the most renowned Neurologist of the USA. Dr. David Perlmutter considers that the use of nutrition to fight and slow the progression of the disease is a remarkable breakthrough, offering hope to those who are struggling with the condition. The Dr. Perlmutter reminds us, "rule number one: You can alter your genetic fate."

Others doctors highlight how the changes in diets across the globe that began in the 60's and 70's are linked to the time that Alzheimer's disease began to rise dramatically, and may be the reason that it continues to rise. In support of this theory, emerging countries that start to adopt an increasingly western-style diet also see an increase in the incidence of Alzheimer's disease. The two doctors Dr. Perlmutter and Dr. Wallach explain that Alzheimer's disease began to become more prevalent after western doctors and health experts started to consider cholesterol and fats as being unhealthy. Saturated fats and cholesterol have been stigmatized to what is described as absurd levels that are associated with overweight and heart disease.

But a diet rich in saturated fats does not contribute to heart diseases in the way that has been thought to be. Researchers from the Harvard School of Public Health conducted a large study recently and came to the conclusion that there is no link between the consumption of high-fat foods and coronary heart illness.

Instead of eating the natural fats in whole food items, we've removed milk and other meat foods of their natural fats, extracting the yolks from eggs, skinless chickens low fat, or non-fat milk, in addition to more artificial methods of taking the fats from our food. Consumption of total fat has dropped to a record low. There's a whole business that produces and markets foods that are low-fat and low-cholesterol which are touted as healthy and 'good for you as simple carbs, gluten and trans-fats have become a staple that we consume in a reckless manner. Even after years of following this diet trend and consuming more calories, obesity levels have never been as high. Heart disease remains the leading reason for deaths. As time passes, Alzheimer's disease is impacting many more people, which is not surprising given that we are constantly depriving our bodies of cholesterol and fat two of the most important components in the brain.

Many doctors have been urging us to shift our attitudes towards fat and cholesterol We must learn to differentiate between the healthy, natural fats that our bodies require and the harmful trans-fats and consider more seriously the dangers of gluten and sugars that are simple consumed. Apart from cholesterol and fats Many nutrients and foods have been linked to brain health. They have also been shown to enhance cognitive function, lessen neural inflammation, and prevent cells from developing typical plaques and tangles associated with Alzheimer's disease. Below are a few of the recommended food items thought by medical professionals to be beneficial for brain health, how they function and the best ways to include them in your diet.

Eggs, Fish Oils and Omega 3

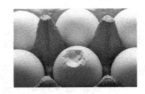

Omega-3 fatty acids can be discovered in nuts, fish, as well as some oils. They can also be consumed as an supplement. Omega-3 fatty acids have been proven for their anti-inflammatory properties and boost the health of the brain. Studies repeatedly show that people who regularly consume fish rich of omega-3 fatty acids such as mackerel, salmon and tuna experience fewer instances that they develop Alzheimer's. Researchers from the National Institutes of

Health support the idea of omega-3 fatty acids could aid in the fight against Alzheimer's disease. There are a variety of fish oil and Omega-3 supplements. Doctor. Fotuhi prescribes his patients to take the DHA fish oil supplement that increases cerebral blood circulation and decreases plaque formation and inflammation. Dr. Fotuhi recommends 600 mg daily. Krill oil is an exclusive kind of omega-3 supplement that is able to neutralize free radicals that are present in your body. It is even thought to block harmful molecules already within the body prior to causing harm.

The majority of omega-3 supplements should be taken along with a fat-rich food in order to be absorbed more effectively into the human body.

Three Essential Supplements: Folic Acid, Vitamin B12 and Vitamin B6

The most frequent ingredients in studies of homeopathy and research are vitamin B6, folic acids and B12. The Dr. David Smith (Oxford University) conducted a study that gave high doses of folic acids B6, B6 and B12 to elderly patients suffering from mild cognitive impairments, who are considered to be at as having a high risk of developing Alzheimer's. When compared to a control group, those who took the vitamins experienced less shrinkage in the entire brain and seven-fold less atrophy areas of the brain more susceptible to damage caused by Alzheimer's. Doctor. Smith announced that the combination of folic acid and vitamin B6 as well as B12 is "the one and only treatment for disease that has proven effective. We've proven that you can alter the symptoms of the disease."

It is crucial to remember it is important to note that vitamin B12 is the most effective when injected since it is not readily taken up by the body, especially for those who are elderly. Doctors typically suggest large doses of B12 in the form of vitamin supplement or suggest sublingual sprays that are more easily absorbed into blood. Dr. Wallach has developed a unique recipe for extremely high doses of vitamin and mineral supplements, which includes of course huge doses of folic acids Vitamin B6, Vitamin B6 as well as vitamin B12 for people suffering from Alzheimer's, by relying on numerous case studies to prove his claim that the condition is curable and ended in a short amount of time.

Essential Spices for Brain Health In this recipe, you will find cinnamon extract and turmeric

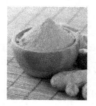

Cinnamon enhances brain function and decreases the formation of plaque within the arteries, resulting in greater blood circulation throughout the body as well as cerebral blood circulation. Cinnamon is also believed to be helpful for memory and the ability to recognize. It is easy to incorporate into your daily diet. You can sprinkle it over your coffee or tea, or flavor cereals, toast oatmeal, toast, or Ice cream, for example.

However, the majority of studies on cinnamon are done using the highest concentration of cinnamon extract which means that you'd need to consume a large amount of cinnamon to achieve similar results. Additionally, the majority of stores sell cinnamon that is not really cinnamon, but rather cassia, another similar plant, which doesn't have similar effects. Real cinnamon is available through specialty stores or online or even by incorporating small quantities of it into your diet can give you health benefits.

Since Alzheimer's is linked with inflammation of the brain on a cell level and cellular level, doctor. Andrew Weil recommends eating turmeric , which is believed as anti-inflammatory. Turmeric aids in helping the body eliminate bad cholesterol, also known as LDL as well as stimulates the brain to produce more antioxidants. Research in mice has shown that a protein found in turmeric can cross the highly sensitive blood-brain barrier (which many drugs are unable to traverse) and prevent plaques from forming (Journal of Food and Agricultural Chemistry). Research suggests some of the main reasons India can boast one of the most low rates of Alzheimer's disease is due to its large intake of turmeric. Turmeric is a mild mustard flavour and turns food items a beautiful yellow. It is a great ingredient to add into curries, teas, or other vegetables such as cauliflower or potatoes, and tastes great sauteed with onions.

Coconut Oil and Other Fats that are Healthy

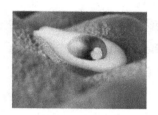

Dr. Mary Newport, supported by Dr. Joseph Mercola, argues that coconut oil could aid in the restoration and renewal of nerve function regardless of whether cells had been damaged. The Dr. Newport explains that the brain requires energy to function and relies on ketones or glucose. Due to today's high-carb, low-sugar diets and problems regarding insulin level, glucose doesn't get to the brain with a consistent supply, leading to neural cells dying and dying. But, the brain could make ketones to help with energy. They are produced by the body by consuming healthy fats, including coconut oil. A diet rich in healthy fats, and low in sugars will encourage the production and utilization of ketones, instead of glucose. The coconut oil can be a nutritious and mildly flavorful oil that is utilized to replace butter or oils. Coconut oil comes with a host of benefits that help protect the brain from damage caused by Alzheimer's disease. For instance , it has been proven to boost the quantity of HDL which is a.k.a. Good Cholesterol, which is essential for a healthy brain function.

Other types of healthy cholesterol that shield brain cells The healthy cholesterol that protects brain cells - HDL are found in poly and monounsaturated fats, such as vegetable and olive oils such as nuts, avocados, and nuts. It is crucial to stay clear of trans-fats that boost bad cholesterol and decrease the good cholesterol. Trans-fats are often listed on nutrition labeling as 'partly hydrogenated oil'.

Antioxidants

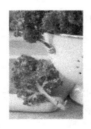

Antioxidants are amazing molecules that have been proven to protect cells from damage within the body. A variety of foods, particularly fruits and vegetables - are abundant in antioxidants. A variety of antioxidants are believed to protect neurons from damage caused by oxidation and Alzheimer's. It is recommended that individuals consume vegetables of all colors to keep a healthy supply of minerals, vitamins, and antioxidants. Superfoods include green leafy vegetables (like spinach and Kale) as well as broccoli and the berries. Berries are especially praised for their ability to combat the loss of memory that is associated with Alzheimer's disease, particularly blueberries from the wild. Doctors suggest drinking a glass of the red or purple variety of grape juice around the time of dinner. Coffee and chocolate are quite beneficial for heart health, and can also have an protection in fighting Alzheimer's. The white, green teas, and oolong have been proved to benefit brain function, they also have anti-inflammatory properties , and contain antioxidants.

Another way to help your body to produce antioxidants is to keep an uninhibited blood sugar levels, as suggested by Dr. Perlmutter. A lower blood sugar level results in less inflammation of the cells which leads to increased levels of antioxidants.

Cholesterol and eggs

Professor. Wallach has provided extensive research that has shown that cholesterol is essential to brain functioning. A cholesterol referred to as Myelin is an important component of the brain , and helps protect neural cells. People with the lowest levels of blood cholesterol suffer significant higher levels of Alzheimer's disease. On the other hand, those with high levels cholesterol - good and bad - perform more on tests of cognitive ability. In the Journals of Biological Chemistry reported that cholesterol and fat found in meat and eggs could actually shield neurons from shrinking or creating Alzheimer's plaques. However, a diet that is low in fat and cholesterol can actually promote neurodegeneration.

The Dr. Wallach encourages a diet that is high in healthy cholesterol and in particular , he recommends an eating plan that is rich in eggs. He suggests that people who are who are at the beginning of Alzheimer's consume 6-8 eggs per day which can be soft-boiled or lightly cooked or scrambled with butter (not oil). He suggests 2 eggs per day as a precautionary measure against Alzheimer's disease. He says it is crucial to keep the yolks soft, so that essential nutrients and fats do not get removed when cooking. He also urges individuals to consume red meats, despite the claims that it causes heart disease.

The importance of Gut Flora

It's not only diet that alters the brain's chemistry however, it is also how the food items are absorbed by the body. Gut bacteria are the main reason for this. The human body needs an essential and intricate array of microbes in the small intestines to process the nutrients and vitamins that are derived from food. It's been widely known that the increasing use of antibiotics, both those prescribed by physicians and the trace present in our food have permanently altered the population's gut bacteria. Just one dose of antibiotics is a huge hazard to the essential bacteria found in the gut. A diet that is high in simple carbs can also alter the gut bacteria and affects the body's ability to absorb nutrients and digest different foods. Fibre is harmful also, since the body creates byproducts from digesting fibres that can be harmful to the gut bacteria.

The gut plays a key role in determining how the food that you consume enter your bloodstream and , consequently, the brain. If your gut is not healthy, you could consume the most healthy food items, but they'll be ineffective because your body won't be able to absorb nutrients. Additionally, bacteria in your gut produce important vitamins such as B12 that are essential to the functioning in the brain.

It's possible that you've lost significant amounts of gut bacteria, which simply will not recover without probiotics. Fortunately, it's never too late to begin treating the our gut the flora. Probiotics supplements are beneficial however, many food items naturally contain large quantities of. Sauerkraut and other fermented vegetables have incredible amounts of beneficial bacteria . even eating small amounts often will provide huge health benefits. Artichokes, kimchiand tempeh, kefir and yoghurt and other vegetables are all excellent ways to keep good probiotic health.

Foods to avoid: Simple Carbs and Gluten

As we have already seen and discussed, there is a consensus with health professionals that gluten and simple carbs can be harmful to the brain and can be extremely harmful to those who are at risk of developing Alzheimer's. Instabil insulin levels and diabetes have been found to damage neurons and hinder the communication between cells, which leads to shrinking of the brain. Doctor. Wallach states that gluten such as barley, wheat, or oats, should be avoided by anyone suffering from a neurological condition. Instabil blood sugar levels can result in damage to brain cells, and they require steady, consistent flow of glucose to function. Additionally, gluten and sugars are extremely harmful to gut floraand can affect the way that the body processes different foods.

Chapter 18: Memory Exercises For The Brain

Memory Exercises

Recent research has altered our knowledge of the brain and revealed its incredible ability to change. Although damage to neurons and the pathways that connect them is thought to be irreparable however, the brain's innate plasticity allows the brain to construct alternative routes around damaged areas , and also utilize healthy neurons to replace damaged ones. The process of plasticity could be the primary factor in resolving cognitive issues and neurodegeneration, in essence slowing the progression of Alzheimer's. Professor. Robert Bender explains with the greatest emphasis that we have to keep working and stimulating our brain in various ways to improve and strengthen neural connections. If we don't do this, our brain's cells begin to weaken and new pathways become more difficult to establish.

The idea that the diagnosis of Alzheimer's disease is essentially the same as the death penalty makes people feel disillusioned, depressed and inactive, and all of these factors can accelerate the process of advancing the illness. This is a serious issue since people are enticed to the illness. Many studies have demonstrated that mental stimulation is effective in slowing the development of Alzheimer's disease or slowing the progression of Alzheimer's during the initial stages that the condition is in its early stages. It is believed that the Longevity Centre at UCLA shows that individuals are more in control of their dementia and Alzheimer's than they think and that with a few simple mental exercises , significant improvement in symptoms is feasible. One study found that among those who suffered from Alzheimer's plaques as well as knots in their brains during post-mortem tests, a third of them maintained normal cognitive function prior to their death.

This shrewd third also had larger hippocampi than other patients who suffered from impairment due to Alzheimer's disease.

The brain's hippocampi is the part that participates in short-term memory generally shrinks by 0.5 percent each year, after the age of 50. But what the Neurexpand Neuro Centre is located in Washington, U.S.A. has demonstrated is that the decline isn't inevitable or 'natural'. Neurexpand has designed a three month treatment plan that involves meditation, cognitive training and fitness exercises, as well as neurofeedback therapy over a period of five hours per week. Most people who take part in the program sees a rise of their hippocampi. This is not just reversed signs of age and loss in memory but actually improving. Some people are successfully reversed 17 years of age.

It is well-known that a more hippocampus is a sign of in less sensitivity to the damage caused by Alzheimer's disease it is apparent that stimulation to the brain is an essential factor in the way that Alzheimer's disease impacts the brain's functioning. This amazing discovery has been verified by UCLA Longevity Centre and extensive research. The physical and mental exercises that these centres suggest are fairly simple and can be performed at your home. They are beneficial to people with early signs of Alzheimer's disease, those who are with a high risk of developing it, and those simply looking to improve their brain health and function. There are many ways to keep yourself busy, active and include more mentally demanding activities into your daily routine What exercises are most effective is different for each person, but some suggestions are offered.

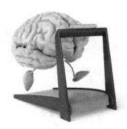

The Dr. Robert Bender recommends mental stimulation by engaging in simple, practical things like reading, engaging in talks, taking part in cards or board games. Brain teasers, crosswords, easy math Sudoku and more all engage and challenge the brain.

Simple memorization exercises such as memorizing cards or a poem, as well as some capital cities in different countries are all fantastic methods to increase the size of your hippocampal. The Dr. Sperling of Neurexpand suggests at least twenty minutes spent on memorization per day. Not enough considering the remarkable increase of memory (with or with Alzheimer's) and possible longevity that just 20 minutes of memorization can bring. The stimulation of the mind can be easily included into everyday activities with having to think about it. Making new dishes can provide an additional benefit, which is making better choices about your diet . It is also an ideal method to stimulate your brain in a variety of ways that require concentration, planning as well as hand-eye coordination. It also stimulates various senses.

Breaking old habits is a great method of engaging your brain for activities you weren't before like eating, brushing your teeth using your hand that is not your dominant one, taking an alternative route to home, or changing the arrangement of your bookcase or furniture in your living space. To take a more thorough method, older people are advised to learn the language of their choice, which is extremely beneficial in preventing the development of dementia. Like learning to play an instrument that is not familiar, or just taking a class (for example, taking classes for adults).

Activities like drawing or knitting can help improve the hand-eye coordination. Another vital aspect of mental fitness is social activities. Social interaction is as an aspect of mental health as exercises for the brain.

Doctors suggest that elderly people attend classes, for example singing or yoga or maybe setting up a reading club with other friends. These classes will be extremely beneficial to the development of cognitive abilities and maintain. Neurofeedback is a revolutionary method that, unfortunately, you can't perform at home. It has however, had remarkable success in improving cognitive function and increasing the capacity that the brain has, and it's a non-invasive method that is fun and enjoyable. Neurofeedback is a method of monitoring the brain's electrical activity and then feeding back the signals to stimulate the creation of new neural connections. Normally, as we age, the strength or speed of brain's electricity (EEG) is reduced and can be observed using a computer that is specially designed for. Neurofeedback detects the regions of the brain with the lowest electrical activity. It provides the patient with various video, music, or images that increase activity in these regions. Research has shown that it can be immensely beneficial, and effectively increase electrical activity in these brain regions.

The long hours spent watching a TV and feeling bored or feeling lonely are all aspects which can lead to brain atrophy. Many elderly suffer from boredom and lack of purpose especially following retirement. Computer games that improve memory - 'brain games' as well as apps designed specifically for those suffering from Alzheimer's disease have been criticized by leading neurologists and doctors of being uneffective in slowing cognitive decline.

Researchers believe that memory boosting games on computers aren't thought to be effective because they don't produce "transfer". In essence playing the game several times can make you more proficient at the game however, it's not much more than this. However, several applications have received favorable reviews, especially Luminosity, Dakim, Clevermind (which is targeted at those who have already been diagnosed with Alzheimer's) as well as Fit brains trainer.

Another key element in promoting the health of your brain is sleep and meditation. Stress can be extremely harmful to the cognitive function and meditation can help clear the mind of the negative influences. Recent research has shown that meditation has been linked to healthier gray material in our brain, especially those in the hippocampal. Sleep deprivation is likely to be an element that contributes to Alzheimer's, as research studies have shown. The theory is that sleeping is essential for the brain's ability to flush of unneeded proteins, especially ones that are located in plaques of Alzheimer's disease, and also in deep sleep, the brain creates and organizes its memories. Sleep disruption can lead to delaying of this essential process of organizing and clearing the brain. This could lead to an increase in the risk of developing Alzheimer's disease.

People who have trouble sleeping need to be evaluated for sleep apnea. They should also develop an established schedule to sleep eight hours each day.

Chapter 19: Physical Activity That Improves

Cognitive Function

According to the Alzheimer's Research & Prevention Foundation claims that regular physical activity will reduce the risk of getting Alzheimer's disease by as much as 50 percent that is an remarkable outcome. A study conducted at The University of Maryland shows that 12 weeks of moderate exercise be a huge boost to neural efficiency, essentially the ability to think more quickly and require less brain activation for every thought. The recommended exercises aren't difficult or exhausting. All exercises that elderly people can perform on their own and easily integrate into their daily routine. The Dr. Carson Smith who was the person who conducted this study declared, "No study has shown that drugs can accomplish what we found to be feasible with exercises." (Newsmax.com; "Exercise can stop Alzheimer's better than Drugs The study") Exercise improves the brain in a variety of ways. It improves circulation of blood, decreasing stress levels and promoting better sleep, increasing your mood, and raising the levels of good cholesterol

114

that is present in your body, while also reducing the amount that are bad cholesterol. In contrast to drugs that are bound to are accompanied by a torrent of negative side effects, and unpredictable long-term impact, exercise has not just proven to improve cognition but it is beneficial for your skin, bones, the heart and lungs, as well as the immune system.

Health professionals and doctors are also of the opinion that exercise is vital to ensure a healthy flow of blood to the brain. This prevents brain damage by enhancing the brain's ability to keep old connections and create new ones. In addition, exercise may reduce the progress of the disease for those who have already begun to experience symptoms. It is crucial to establish the routine of exercise as early as possible.

People with Alzheimer's tend to neglect exercises and can quickly fall into a sedentary state in their lives. For those who are at risk or at risk of developing Alzheimer's disease is a mix of strength training, in addition to relaxation exercises such as yoga, meditation, Pilates, or deep breathing.

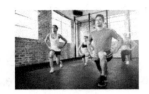

Stress levels that are excessive and low mental stimulation are associated with cognitive decline and dementia. The effects of stress upon the mind is quite alarming which is why, when stress levels increase across the country the rate of dementia is increasing. Yoga, exercise as well as meditation are vital to help manage stress. All forms of yoga, meditation, Pilates, or deep breathing exercises have been proven to calm the mind and ease stress, and result in more restful sleep. Neuroscientist Dr. Helen Lavretsky points out the ways yoga can stimulate different areas of the brain. It includes breathing, movements that balance, coordination various movements such as chanting, visualization and concentration. It's a different way to stimulate your brain to establish new connections as well as strengthen existing ones.

In addition, the stress-reducing aspect of yoga is crucial for cognition and memory. People suffering from Alzheimer's disease are at a high chance of suffering injuries from falls that lead to them becoming bedridden or sedentary. Seniors should be mindful when exercising and keep in mind that head injuries are believed to trigger dementia. Being in good condition means that you are less prone to accidents and falls that happen in your everyday activities. Exercise helps improve balance, strength , and flexibility, but it is crucial that exercise isn't overly strenuous, and performed under the supervision of a professional or security. Studies conducted from University of Washington researchers University of Washington found that those with higher stability were 3 times more likely develop dementia. Balance naturally declines as we age, and people become more difficult to maintain their balance. There are many exercises which can aid in improving balance, such as yoga and tai-chi. One simple, but highly effective way to exercise is to sit with one foot for 30 minutes at a stretch however this should be done in a safe manner to ensure you don't hurt yourself should you fall.

Doctors advise combining aerobics and strengthening exercises to maximize the effect. Aerobic exercise has been proven to boost mental and physical capacities. Walking for walks or engaging in exercises like yoga Pilates and tai the chi are suggested, however dependent on your physical ability and fitness level, more vigorous activities such as swimming can be beneficial. A walk that is vigorous has many benefits apart from general health. Walking outside lets you breathe in the fresh air, other people, as well as different sights as well as sounds and scents. Yoga is a great choice because it requires different types of exercises and demands constant training and mental exercise instead of merely routine movements that do not stimulate your brain, and can be accomplished in the help of a group. The recommended amounts of exercise for those in the beginning stages of Alzheimer's are similar to the amounts suggested for people who are elderly 150 minutes moderately vigorous workouts per week. This is difficult enough to work up a sweat, yet you can still engage in an engaging conversation during the exercise. Things like gardening and cleaning are also aerobic activities.

Three to four sessions of strength training per week is suggested for better balance and to keep muscles mass. This can help in strengthening bones and reducing their fragility. Regular exercise in the strength area was found in studies to help improve the daily tasks like taking stairs, walking and putting on clothes and other minor but crucial everyday activities that give those with Alzheimer's such difficulty. Dr. Fotuhi suggests push-ups as the ideal exercise for those suffering from Alzheimer's disease. According to him, it's an easy endurance and resistance exercise for the brain. It increases blood flow throughout the body. It doesn't require any equipment of any kind, and is virtually impossible to be injured during. Five to seven push-ups each day is enough to see a significant improvement in your mental health.

The Alzheimer's Research and Prevention Foundation recommends that people, specifically those who are at risk of developing Alzheimer's, or those who are who are in the beginning stages of the disease, to perform the 12 minutes of yoga known as Kirtan Kriya which has the potential to reduce stress and increase the activity of the hippocampus in the brain. Kirtan Kriya is a practice for hundreds of years. The specific movements are beneficial for coordination, and the notes are thought to connect areas in the roof of the mouth that connect to brain cells. The meditation practice is performed by having open eyes and with a bent spine. It involves drawing the energy from at the top of your head, and from the middle of your forehead. The technique involves touching the point of each finger with the thumbs of each hand, and then gently singing the mantra "Saa Taa, Naa Maa'. Kirtan Kriya is a specific exercise that has been found to be significantly more effective over other types of meditation that are used to treat Alzheimer's disease.

Acupuncture is also proven to decrease anxiety and stress. People suffering from Alzheimer's disease who were treated regularly with acupuncture during Hong Kong demonstrated improvements in the ability to communicate, cognition motor skills, as well as cognition.

More studies are currently underway to verify the efficacy of acupuncture for treating other behavioural and mood disorders. Massage, too, has been shown to provide numerous therapeutic benefits and even in reducing irritation, wandering and aggression in those suffering from Alzheimer's.

Chapter 20: Cognitive Disorders 101

Both Alzheimer's disease and dementia are regarded as cognitive disorders, and therefore they need to be treated. This chapter will concentrate on explaining them as well as the signs and medical procedures to be used to determine their cause.

Do they differ from one another?

One of the most common misconceptions people face about Alzheimer's is same as dementia. In reality, they're both classified as cognitive conditions. In order to be able to answer this question, a thorough explanation of both of them first is crucial.

Dementia

In accordance with the Fourth Text Revised Edition of the Diagnostic and Statistical Manual for Mental Disorders A person may be diagnosed with dementia If the following signs are present in the person:

A. There is a possibility of the development of a number of cognitive deficiencies which are apparent in two symptoms:

1. Memory impairment The person finds it difficult to recall information already exists or is having difficulty when learning new information.

2. A few or all of these cognitive problems could be a sign of cognitive disturbances:

A. Language impairment (aphasia regardless of kind)

b. difficulty in performing motor tasks regardless of whether the person is able to perform motor activities normally (apraxia)

C. A difficulty in sensing or recognizing objects despite the fact that they have normal sensory functions (agnosia)

D. Instability with executive functioning, like abstracting, organizing and making plans

B. Criteria A1 and A2 cause significant impairments in the person's occupational and social functioning. Also, there is an apparent reduction in their current performance.

C. The symptoms shouldn't be an indirect or direct cause of any general or mental health condition.

Alzheimer's disease

This condition is diagnosed when the conditions mentioned above are observed by a person, but there are a few additional criteria:

* The beginning of the illness is gradual and the decline in cognition is expected to continue;

* The age at which this condition may manifest will be 65. those who suffer from it prior to or after this age are identified as having an the condition with an early or late onset Alzheimer's, respectively.

Simply stated, Dementia consists of a vast array of cognitive diseases that include Alzheimer's condition as one of its forms. They might be alike in that those with Alzheimer's disease are thought to be suffering from dementia (since it is an aspect of the latter). The fact is that Alzheimer's is by far the most common kind of dementia. The difference between them is the fact that dementia may have different forms and is triggered by different situations. But Alzheimer's disease is caused by dementia, and does not possess any other forms.

How do they get diagnosed?

The person's loss of memory and other signs that are a result of dementia could be due to various factors. Therefore it is important that the person be prepared to undergo a several tests to determine that the problem is really due to dementia. In addition to looking over their medical records doctors may also perform these tests

a. Brain scans: The patient will go through an array of tests that provide the doctor an image of the brain of the patient. By analyzing the results, doctors can determine if the organ has been physically damaged due to stroke or bleeding or to determine whether there is any tumor. A few of these tests are computerized (CT) and Postron emission Tomography (PET) scans as well as Magnetic resonance imaging (MRI).

B. Neuropsychological and cognitive examinations are designed to assess the person's cognitive (thinking) abilities. This includes a range of tests designed to assess different abilities like attention, judgment and reasoning as well as language abilities (grammar as well as vocabulary) as well as memory and their general orientation. In this way they are able to identify if a sufferer has the condition and the severity of it, and identify which brain region is affected.

C. Lab tests - this can eliminate any possibility that signs of dementia are due to physical issues that affect the brain's functioning. A few of them include hypothyroidism or vitamin deficiencies.

d. Neurological assessment - This test is a way to test the individual's mobility, balance and senses, reflexes as well as other areas that affect the functioning of their brain. This test can be used to determine the cause of the symptoms.

e. A psychiatric assessment - meeting an appointment with a health specialist like a psychologist or psychiatrist can assist in determining if the issue is caused by other psychological issues, such as depression. They may also conduct interviews with family members and acquaintances to determine if there is a decline in the patient's performance prior to the assessment.

Knowing the signs of the condition and understanding the procedure that must be followed to make an accurate diagnosis is essential. When they are aware of these basic facts, people will be able to determine whether they (or anyone they consider to be their loved relatives) suffer from the disorder. This can help in the development of a more appropriate treatment and treatment program.

Chapter 21: Taking Care Of What Your Doctor Prescribed Learn What Treatments And Medications Are Prescribed For Dementia And Alzheimer's.

To date there hasn't been a method to treat these disorders even though their causes were previously identified. But, the majority of doctors suggest various treatments to manage the symptoms that are caused by the condition.

Medical Interventions

Below is a brief description of medical treatments that are offered to patients who are diagnosed for the purpose of reducing the progress of the disease. Also included are the adverse effects of each.

1. Donepezil Galantamine Donepezil, Galantamine and Rivastigmine All of these generics are called cholinesterase inhibitors and their goal is to raise the levels of a certain chemical messenger within the body responsible for improving judgment and memory. In addition to Alzheimer's and Dementia (even its different types) It is also used to treat Parkinson's disease.

Patients, however, could experience the following adverse effects when the use of these inhibitors

* Diarrhea

* Nausea

* Vomiting

2. Memantine regulates glutamate levels in our body Another chemical messenger could affect some of our brain's functions, including memory and learning. When using this drug patients may feel dizzy. Certain researchers have suggested that this drug, in conjunction with any other cholinesterase inhibitor will yield better results than using them separately.

3. The purpose of occupational therapy is done with the intention of helping patients adapt to their conditions. They are taught adaptive behaviors. In that way they are able to carry on with their daily tasks without being hindered by the changes they'll eventually face.

4. Other medications that can treat other symptoms or conditions that an individual may be experiencing.

Non-medical intervention

Apart from the ones recommended by medical professionals, there are modifications that could be beneficial to people with the disease, such as:

1. The environment in which the patient lives by reducing distractions like noise and clutter could assist them in staying focused and less confused and annoyed.

2. Breaking down tasks into simple steps due to the declining cognitive abilities of the patient they might find a variety of complex instructions hard to understand and may cause frustration. Family members or caregivers may be able to assist the patient's direction by being attentive to them while they complete each step at each step. This can help them adjust to the new way of doing things (eventually becoming habitual) and also assist them in continuing contributing to the family.

The assistance of experts in geriatric health can not only assist the patient, but assist the family with what they can do to help to improve the health of the person who is affected. In the end, you can't depend on medical treatment.

Chapter 22: Reduce The Chance Of Developing The Disease Changes In Lifestyle Can Assist In Preventing The Development Dementia And Alzheimer's

Prevention is always more effective than treatment. While every function in the human body are bound to diminish with time however, it is not the case that these diseases are not part of the natural process. But, there are certain ways to practice to follow that (although not a guarantee to avoid contracting the condition) can reduce the chance of developing these. According to research, those who practice these practices have a lower risk of being affected by the disorder. In this chapter, these habits will be reviewed.

Build your social connections

Humans are social beings, and most people cannot think of surviving without the assistance of someone else. Being connected to other people is beneficial for the brain. According to research that people who spend a lot of time with family and friends are more successful in memory and cognition as opposed to those who spend less time with their friends. This is why the social life of a person should be an important factor.

As a person gets older and gets older, their time spent with others is drastically diminished, which can be detrimental to the brain. Therefore, it is crucial to be connected and develop connections. You can accomplish this through these methods:

A social gathering such as senior centers is among the best ways to form connections. Many towns have societies that collect the senior citizens of their area and arrange events specifically for them. This is particularly beneficial to those suffering from"empty nest syndrome" (situation that parents feel sadness as all their children have left their home to create family of their own). Additionally, they are able connect with new friends (aside from the ones they had in their earlier times) that can act as an emotional support group due to their shared experiences. This also allows them to keep active. The fact that they're older does not mean they can't accomplish anything.

* Connect with old friends by attending an ongoing meeting or social media - networking isn't just about getting to meet individuals in

132

person. Plan a time to meet them every few months (annually and quarterly perhaps even monthly) and continue to connect with them via non-personal methods such as e-mails, telephones, or even through networking websites such as Facebook. Being informed about them means that you must remember important events they've shared with you, thereby improving your memory and recall.

* Going to public spaces like parks can also be a way of getting to know more people, apart from being aware of changes taking place in their area.

• Finding something they love doing together or doing something different even if one does not find joy in going out or getting to know people outside of their comfort area, they may still reconnect with old acquaintances by engaging in activities that they love doing together, or even try something different. This could make the relationship more enjoyable and stronger.

Exercise regularly

This is one habit that one should be able to be able to develop no matter their age. Apart from the obvious benefits to physical fitness and fitness, research suggests that those who regularly exercise have a lower chance of developing Alzheimer's disease and dementia, which can reduce it by up to 50.

What should be included in their exercise program?

While older individuals may struggle to exercise in the same way that younger people can do however, there are some activities thought of as exercise that are feasible for them due to their age.

* Aerobic exercises - - these are all exercises which increases the heart rate of the participant. While in gym workouts is implying that one exercise on a treadmill or run around the neighborhood, people who are older can still achieve the same results by performing certain routine tasks such as walking briskly or cleaning up the house and even gardening. If they are looking for an easier form fitness, they could add swimming to their daily routine. It is suggested that this kind of exercise should be performed every week five times.

Training for strength and endurance These are exercises designed to build muscle. It was observed that building mass when combined with aerobics is more effective than doing them both on their own. If you are over 65years old, it is recommended to talk to your doctor about specific positions that can be accomplished and also advise their weight limit that they can train using during their workout. It is suggested that this workout routine is repeated every 2 to 3 days per week.

Chapter 23: Becoming Aware Of Your Food Choices A List Of Foods That Can Help Improve Your Mind

Another thing that needs to be implemented to lower the risk of developing these disorders is to incorporate foods with ingredients that aid in the health of the brain. This chapter will discuss these food items and their components and advantages will be discussed.

1. The leafy greens of vegetables like mustard, collard, kale and spinach contain folate and vitamins B9, ingredients that can aid in the reduction of depression and help improve cognitive function.

2. The berries are high of Vitamins C as well as E (boosts immunity and are beneficial for skin health as well) Every variety of berries contain anthocyanin. This substance is known to shield the brain from harm that could result from free radicals within the body.

3. Beans, in addition to their folate in this food, it (as along with legumes) includes magnesium, potassium as well as iron. These elements help to

improve general health and enhances the firing of neurons (so that nerve impulses are sent to the brain more quickly which triggers a more rapid reaction). The foods also help increase the neurotransmitter acetylcholine that may affect the brain's functions.

4. Cruciferous vegetables such as broccoli Brussels sprouts and Chinese cabbages also contain folate, which can reduce homocysteine levels (a component that can trigger neurological disorders like mental impairments).

5. A variety of nuts like cashews, almonds hazelnuts and peanuts walnuts, and pecans have various components that aid for brain functions of anyone. They contain folate, magnesium, as well as omega 3 and 6.

6. Vegetables like asparagus beets and carrots tomatoes, and squash are all known to be rich in Vitamin A iron, Vitamin A, and folate. These are components that aid in improving cognition.

7. Both are considered natural supplements that provide your body with omega-3 fats. Based on some studies that were conducted, it was discovered that this ingredient can lower the risk of developing lesion on the brain by about 26

percent since damage to the brain could cause conditions to develop.

8. Seeds of sunflower and pumpkin - could be considered an appropriate food source for your pet's hamster however, these seeds are loaded with the choline (component which can increase the amount of Acetylcholine) as well as zinc (known to boost the memory and cognition of a person).

9. Coconut oil is a source of ingredients that aid in eliminating amyloids within the brain, a damaging component that can lead to neurodegenerative diseases like the Alzheimer's disease and other dementias. In addition it also aids in the make ketones, which is a chemical which helps breakdown glucose within the brain.

10. Turmeric is a different food ingredient which is also known to rid the brain of amyloids. It is among the most commonly used ingredients in curry as well as in the majority of meals eaten by people who live in India. Therefore, the small number of people suffering from Alzheimer's or dementia in the country could be due to their diet.

11. Eggs that are produced by pastured chicken
The eggs that are produced by chickens permitted to roam freely were discovered to have higher levels of Vitamin B12 and omega 3 acid fatty acids, both of them are essential elements that help maintain the health of your brain.

12. Cinnamon - the most commonly used ingredient in the kitchen is known to have compounds that stop the growth in brain cells. Another study found that the smell of it can enhance a person's cognitive abilities and memory. But, anyone who wants to drink cinnamon must be aware that consuming the spice in large quantities can cause a rise in heart rate. It can also cause sleepiness and depression. It can also lead to skin and oral lesions.

13. Certain fish species like salmons and sardines contain omega 3 acid, but includes other ingredients which are beneficial to well-being. It is calcium (for bone density) and ferrous (good for the red blood cell that provide oxygen to all regions of the body, including the brain) as well as magnesium (ensures the proper functioning of nerves) as well as potassium (known to enhance neuron transmission impulses) and B vitamins.

Food is among the major sources of energy for our bodies. Therefore, knowing the ingredients that a particular food is essential for building a stronger immunity to any illness, which includes cognitive diseases.

Chapter 24: The Natural Approach Of The Prevention And Treatment Of Alzheimer's Disease.

North American society has spent lots of time and energy as well as funds on research that explores the changes that occur to the human body as we get older. These findings may be disappointing and the dangers are growing for coronary disease, as well as the other normal signs of ageing'. But these aren't the only things that research has discovered!

Take a look at what the past century has brought to longevity We are now living two (and often three) times longer than we were once expected to live to 90s, and even beyond! This is fantastic, but it also raises the possibility of dementia being able to be a reality (in every way).

The best part is there's steps you can take to prevent the onset of dementia, or even Alzheimer's disease. If you are able to make a conscious effort to eat healthy as well as being active and generally aiming to be (and be) well, you'll be well on the path to enjoying the happy healthy old age we all want.

It's crucial to acknowledge the role on the mental side of a healthy aging. It's more than your body. The mind requires just as much assistance to maintain its health and well-being as the body however, it is often ignored. This guide will provide a brief overview of the way that the brain comes in the process of preventing and management of the disease disease, and help you understand the processes taking place inside your body. This guide will provide you with tips for better health, both mentally and physically.

I'll be focusing on explaining more than the physical aspects of Alzheimer'sdisease, since there's more to learn about it. Alzheimer's affects the body but it also affects the mind and can affect our social life as well as our general feeling of well-being. Our families and friends are also affected by Alzheimer's This is why it's important to to do everything you can to stay well-maintained - keeping the suffering of your loved ones to a minimum , as well as to enable you to keep your social life, as well as your mental and physical health.

Everything worthwhile to do is worthwhile if done correctly I'm going to suggest that doing things right starts with formulating an action plan. The plan that this guide will help you begin is to improve your health by teaching you the fundamentals of caring for both your body and mind.

I've included an idea of a 30-day plan This is not intended to be a lifestyle change guide.

Last but not least, I would like to assure you. Anyone could take this book in and gain from it. No matter if you're aged 22 , 67, or even 22 you need to be working to improve your mental health!

Where did we discover Alzheimer's Disease?

Alzheimer's first became known as an illness in 1907 because of the work by Alois Alzheimer.

Alois Alzheimer (go figure). He was conducting an autopsy of a person and discovered tangled neurons in her brain, which was one of the symptoms of Alzheimer's. Incredibly curious as an authentic scientist is often the Dr. Alzheimer investigated the tangles and the resulting Alzheimer's plaque as well as published the findings on the heading of "pre-senile dementia" in a reputable medical journal of the time.

In the period of time it was normal for aging to be a path toward senility, which is the loss of one's brain and ability to recall things or care for oneself. The doctor described this woman's condition to be "pre-senile dementia" since, although she was slowing losing her strength, she was only 51 years old, making the time of onset unpredictable and the reason for recognition.

Today we can detect the onset of Alzheimer's Disease (AD), and recognize that not everyone suffers from it, but the incidences of Alzheimer's disease are increasing. Recent research has revealed that there are 4.5 million people suffering from Alzheimer's Disease in America which is an increase by 2.25 million in 1960.

The positive side is that because of Dr. Alzheimer's research and the efforts of a lot of others who have followed we can now detect Alzheimer's disease and are trying to prevent it from occurring.

This book will examine the evidence and let you know tested and proven methods to aid the people you cherish.

Alzheimer's isn't yet a cure however we can do our best to treat it before we understand the root of what that has caused it.

What is Alzheimer's Disease?

Alzheimer's is an disease that affects the brain's abilities, particularly affecting focus on memory. The symptoms manifest as a failure to care for oneself (forgetting that you switched the stove on , which could cause fire and then forgetting where you're at and then getting lost) without supervision or assistance.

However, there has been no treatment for the disease, however, there are methods to manage the signs and allow patients to lead more of a normal life than was previously believed. Treatment of the signs of AD will increase the life span of the patient, reduce stress of taking care

144

of a beloved one's relatives and friends and improve living quality of the person diagnosed.

Incredibly, there isn't a specific method to diagnose Alzheimer's until the time of death, in the autopsy. This is due to the fact that the signs of Alzheimer's disease are usually hidden deep in the brain in the form of plaque build-ups and neural tangles. ups. However, this doesn't hinder us from trying, however.

When it is discovered that Alzheimer's disease is a possibility that it is a possibility, doctors begin conducting scientific tests to detect the symptoms that typically associated with Alzheimer's. Treatment and diagnosis usually begins when we notice signs and symptoms. However, it's more beneficial to prepare for AD before the signs are evident.

How do we accomplish that? Neural imaging.

Alzheimer's starts to shift its hand during the years prior to the appearance of symptoms. For certain people, the signs begin to manifest as early as 40. However, for others, symptoms may not show up until in their 80s or beyond. The goal is to spot these symptoms in your mind as soon as it is possible to begin treatment earlier rather than later, since it's always the easiest decision to make.

What is the difference between Alzheimer's and Dementia?

Many people become confused from time moment between dementia and Alzheimer's. Both of these conditions can affect memory, and both can lead to the loss of independence needing full-time care after the beginning.

Disorders that have symptoms similar to Alzheimer's

* Depression
* Hypothyroidism
* The Lou Gehrig's disease
* Malnutrition
* Parkinson's disease
* Stroke
* Subdural Hematoma (bleeding within the brain)
* Substance abuse
* Tumors

The misdiagnosis is not uncommon If you keep in mind the symptoms of the patient and then contacting an expert physician, you can reduce the chance of being diagnosed. Medical professionals are aware of the connection between these health concerns, and they are aware of what makes them different and, consequently, what to look for in a diagnosis.

Therefore, the best method to ensure that you or a loved ones are appropriately cared for is to keep track of the symptoms and consult a medical professional in the event that you suspect Alzheimer's disease to be the cause of the changes.

The process of identifying Alzheimer's

Alzheimer's needs to be tested to determine the cause as well as cannot be completely diagnosed until death, however medical professionals are largely adept at determining whether an individual is suffering from Alzheimer's.

To be able to predict this, however, the patient needs to go to a testing facility. This is a challenge for those suffering from Alzheimer's disease, since they typically suffer from) decline in memory (making it more difficult to keep appointments and schedule them) as well as b) anxiety about the appearance in their signs.

There's no reason for you to feel embarrassed in the event that you believe that you or someone you care about, suffers from Alzheimer's disease! There is no need to be ashamed! The most important thing is to speak to the person with compassion or speak with your family and friends to find out what they think regarding the possibility of being diagnosed with Alzheimer's disease and the signs that you are experiencing.

In this chapter will review some of the more easily identified symptoms for patients with Alzheimer's in order to make it simpler for you or your loved one to determine whether Alzheimer's disease is working.

Get tested if you believe you be suffering from Alzheimer's disease - self diagnosis is not acceptable! !

The Alzheimer's symptom checklist:

• Does this person have difficulty with daily tasks that were not a problem for them?

* Is the person appearing older and more exhausted lately?

Are the individual's attention being affected, or perhaps resulting with difficulty during conversations or paying attention to an activity?

* Are they more confused, in particular in areas that don't seem to make sense for the person?

Do you feel that people are often having trouble finding the right words to use?

* Are they taking a break from social life and social activities?

These are the kinds of behaviors you may observe in your family members, friends and, sometimes, even within your own. If you're responding to more than two or three the above questions, it might be time to find an opinion from a doctor. Keep in mind that even if you don't have Alzheimer's that is causing your brain to be troubled there could be something else that needs to be checked out!

The progression of Alzheimer's - - Stages to Look Out for

Alzheimer's, just like all diseases is a process that goes through phases. This chapter will outline the common stages of Alzheimer's disease so that you are able to recognize these in yourself and your loved family members.

What's going on inside the body

The formal stages off the table first. You won't be able recognize these stages, but they can assist you in understanding what's happening to your loved ones. We will then look at the stages that are informal - they are the ones you'll most likely be able to identify.

Stage 1. Lesions

What is it that it appears to look like?

* Lesions appear and begin to cause injury to the brain's entorhinal cortex (in your head, but not apparent).

There is no reason to worry at this point In fact, you won't even be able recognize any visible signs yet as the damage to the brain is only just getting started.

What is the duration of this stage? The initial stage is long-lasting and may last between 10 and 50 years prior to progressing.

Stage 2. Endangering damage to the hippocampus

What does it look like?

* The result of decades of lesioning has led to brain damage in the present particularly in the hippocampal region (a section in the cortex of the entorhinal).

* Memory loss that is short-term symptoms begin to manifest.

The hippocampus plays a role in memory, which is why you see the manifestation of the symptoms clearly. It is at this point that you can start to observe memory impairment at the very least for short-term tasks or tasks, and it could also be mood changes, for example. the regulation of mood (as the hippocampus is also thought to play an important role within this).

How long does it last? This stage lasts between two to four years.

Stage 3. Spreading

What is it that it appears to look like?

* The lesions which began at the level of the entorhinal cortex are expanding throughout the brain and affecting other brain regions.

* Symptoms are apparent right today.

As the damage increases the appearance of signs are growing. Then, Alzheimer's lesions will hit the brain areas that are used to understand the familiar, connect concepts as well as to formulate new concepts.

This is among the most difficult stages because it's the moment when the family members are 'forgotten'.

How long does this last? The duration of this stage is anywhere between 2 and 8 years.

Stage 4. Moderate dementia

What is it that it appears to look like?

* Muscle pains

* Bouts of bizarre behaviour

* Paranoia

This stage is when there is a spread of lesions and plaques to the frontal lobe the brain that is responsible for perception and good judgement and reasoning. This is the reason you notice symptoms like irrational behavior and paranoia or muscle discomforts. The brain is being played by the brain to cause these symptoms.

Everyone has seen it that they are experiencing symptoms by now. The patient might even be misdiagnosed as having dementia.

What is the duration of this stage? The stage can last between two to six years.

Stage 5. The last stages of Alzheimer's disease.

What does it look like?

* Extreme dementia

* Inability to take care of oneself

• Health issues that are frequent due to breakdowns of communication

What is the duration of this stage? This stage usually lasts from two and four years.

It is the last phase of Alzheimer's disease, and like the name implies it usually is the end for the person. At this point the patient is incapable of taking care of themselves in any way, may be showing irrational behavior and may be at a higher risk of health problems - and will be unable to explain the issues they are experiencing in their internal world to receive the appropriate medical treatment.

Now, we will spend some time examining the less obvious signs of Alzheimer's disease, since you might be unable to detect "brain damage" until it's way too late to offer assistance.

Stages of informality

Stage 1. Memory issues

What does it look like?

* Having trouble remembering things that aren't just routine tasks (car keys and what you were up to, etc.)

You may lose the track of where you are

* Often being unable to recall names, locations and so on.

This is typically when misdiagnosis takes place. A few of the things that Alzheimer's is incorrectly diagnosed with are hormonal changes, or mental health problems that result in hormone imbalances (like depression).

153

On the other side of this, often this phase is ignored, or thought of as "just becoming older". The patient is capable of speaking, even when they forget the words they're trying reference. The ability to comprehend is intact However, recall is beginning to fall off here.

The signs we mentioned above are normal indicators of normal memory lapses however, a greater frequency or intensity of your forgetting could be a sign of a problem and needs to be evaluated.

Stage 2. The moment when others begin to panic. What is it that it appears to look like?

* Repeating oneself over and over

* Breaking communication down into sentences in fragments

* Some self awareness, potential for social embarrassment/depression

It is here that people start to worry. You might be repeating yourself, asking the same question to people or needing to be explained things differently, but you cannot seem to figure it out.

Communication skills start to fail at this point. It's because you're trying not only to recall the right word however, you also need to understand the meaning behind what you're trying say. The person begins to speak in terms, saying things such as "where is the material we use to cover food leftovers" in place of "where is the plastic wrap".

This can lead to social isolationas it is a goal by the person who is suffering in order to avoid the shame of being viewed in a negative light as "crazy" and "senile". This can be evident in the fact that people close to you may start to notice changes in your behavior, and could be worried about them and voice their anxiety.

This stage could last for a while before the patient decides to seek medical attention, so be on the lookout for this as the subsequent stages will be much more serious.

Advanced Stages:

The progressions upwards from two indicate an increase in tendency to forget, and most frighteningly - the inability to comprehend the issues that others are noticing. This is why the Alzheimer's patient will often claim their case that they're "fine" to manage themselves, while caregivers who are ill-equipped must fight them to get treatment.

In the last phases of the disease patients may not be able to grasp the basics of understanding (like days and nights). They might revert back to a state of peace or joy in the past and believe that it was a long time ago. The changes can affect the person's ability to locate themselves (or navigate) and could cause a lot of anxiety for family members wondering if their loved ones will be able to be able to find their way back to home. The patient's experience leaves them completely unaware of what's happening. Patients often find themselves in areas they don't have comprehension or memory of.

In the end, the individual is likely to be unable communicate effectively. This could cause many medical issues due to the fact that the patient is unable to convey at the minimum information about dehydration or the source of infection, and so on. In the end, Alzheimer's is a common cause to kill patients with a different health issue which the patient is incapable of explaining to their doctors.

This is when full-time surveillance of the patient is required, and it can be a difficult pill to swallow for people affected. The more advanced stages of

Alzheimer's disease can cause depression, irritability as well as other signs that the patient may feel they're not getting the treatment they were used to be - but cannot understand why.

If a person is at the levels where they are not able to take care of themselves and struggle to communicate, the typical life expectation is 2.5 additional years after this point. This can be due to a range of reasons and is a function of an average.

Conclusions:

As we can see from our timelines Alzheimer's is actually an ongoing disease. One of the benefits is that the person you love may live long enough after being diagnosed However there is a long-lasting harm that living with Alzheimer's causes.

Potential causes of Alzheimer's

Before we discuss the causes of Alzheimer's disease it is important to make it clear that scientists aren't sure regarding this. Research has been conducted for many years and, to date, most of the things we have identified as the causes are physical symptoms. Beyond the signs that trigger the damage the only thing we are aware of is that something is responsible for the development of Alzheimer's.

In terms of physiology is Alzheimer's the cause? The neuron tangles that develop these tangles permit the formation of plaque which can weaken and cause damage to connections within the brain.

What are some theories we've thought of to explain the cause of Alzheimer's disease? Let's have a look:

* Theorem of Aluminum Alongside the notorious plaques and tangles that are characteristic of the brains of people suffering from Alzheimer's Additionally, there is an over-the-top amount of aluminum located in. Some people have begun to believe that aluminum could be linked to the development of Alzheimer's.

This theory has even led some to change anti-antiperspirants, believing the aluminum content to be too high - and that it may build up over time.

The poison is Mercury. Long-term exposure to mercury may be the cause for Alzheimer's disease.

* Deficiencies in nutrition (often Vitamins A & E, acetylcholine, and zinc are thought to be the cause) It is common to examine our diets to find out what is causing the health issues we face and Alzheimer's research is not any different. It could be that a nutrient insufficientity could trigger the production of a chemical which causes plaque and tangles.

* Protein, specifically in particular, specifically, the Alzheimer's Disease Associated Protein (ADAP). The protein was found following autopsy, however, scientists speculate that if could find a way to recognize it before the time of dying, maybe we could intervene to determine if it's actually the primary cause.

A virus aren't just a matter of infecting your PCs, researchers have speculated that the disease could possibly be caused by viruses that we aren't aware of.

Does Genetics Play A Role In Alzheimer's?

The previous chapter discussed several of the popular neurological theories on what causes Alzheimer's disease, but what's the truth about genetics? If you aren't aware, genetics is an expression used to describe your genes, or the pieces of DNA that you receive from your parents during the time of conception.

DNA functions as a blueprint that make up your body. It contains the "plans" for everything from your eye color to height. It can frequently indicate risk for diseases and more.

Genetics are a factor in the development a variety of health issues, and possibly even behavioral problems However, are they playing an important role in the development of Alzheimer's disease?

Researchers are extremely cautious about the things they discuss about this. In this article, I will summarise the findings from the study and discuss the implications

* People suffering from Alzheimer's earlier in life are more likely to be affected by abnormalities on the chromosomes 1,14, and 21.

* People suffering with Alzheimer's disease later in life are more likely to be affected by abnormalities on the 19th chromosome and the development of Apoliprotein E (apoE).

It is very rare to find a family association with Alzheimer's, which means that the if a relative in your family is suffering from Alzheimer's, you're 10 percent more likely to develop it.

The findings don't reveal much but there are lessons we can take from these findings.

1. The odds are only 10% for a chance of having a genetic link. This is extremely low and suggests that the impact of the environment is greater than the influence of your genes on whether or not you'll be diagnosed with Alzheimer's disease.

2. Protein is implicated in the process of developing Alzheimer's however, we don't know what it is.

The reality is that research indicates that lifestyle and environmental choices play a greater impact than family history in Alzheimer's, yet family history may play an important role at times.

This article will go through some of the ways that you could do in order to decrease your riskand also the risk factors. It is interesting to note that nicotine is just one of the risk factors! Nicotine is known to improve memory but it also damages other areas of the brain, transforming the way an Alzheimer's sufferer experiences Alzheimer's drastically (initially to improve however, eventually to the negative)!

Treating Alzheimer's

Alzheimer's is considered a chronic disease that has no cure. The science community is always working in the direction of becoming able to prevent Alzheimer's completely or eliminate it, however, for now we've only found a few signs of the issue and potential solutions to treat these symptoms.

In this way, while keeping the signs and symptoms the medical profession moves to treat Alzheimer's disease as well as they can.

This chapter will go over some of the commonly used treatments for Alzheimer's. Then, we'll look at some organic remedies you can try, as well as some lifestyle choices you could take, however for this moment, we'll focus on medications.

There are many medications we employ to treat Alzheimer's and we'll go over each one. They have been successful in extending people's independence and improving their the quality of living. This is the great news.

Incidious Side Effects

The downside is that these medicines can have adverse effects and you must be aware of these. Estimates vary, but the current estimations suggest that up to 20% of people taking

Alzheimer's drugs experience at least one major adverse effect.

What are the typical side effects that can be triggered by using medications?

* Aches

* Diarrhea

* Heartburn

* An increase in aggression possible because you've regained the awareness of the world in the world around you. You begin to become annoyed with the condition completely and express it in your daily behavior however the main point is that aggression can be a consequence.

* Nausea, vomiting

* Other rare adverse effects

We also included the class "other rare, uncommon adverse effects" in order to emphasize the fact that sometimes medication can cause different effects on people of different. All of us are unique and how our bodies react to the drugs can have a lot to do with our physical and mental reactions to these drugs.

Extreme side effects

* Variation in frequency and volume of urine

* Sudden seizure (particularly where seizures were not present before)

* Slowed pulse

* Eyes with jaundice (yellowing)

Beware: If any of the above symptoms occur when you start taking a medication, inform your doctor be aware immediately! It is not advisable to take any risks when you experience these symptoms, because they are connected to more serious health conditions and problems.

Medical attention is a must to stop many of the unpleasant adverse effects right away.

Medicines

In this regard, we're going to go over the medication itself. You are welcome to use the chapter for reference Returning for more details.

Possibility of Multiple Medication

Take note that while dealing with Alzheimer's disease the patients are looking to treat many symptoms. This may lead to various medications, perhaps one to treat symptoms of the disease as well as others to address the potential negative effects of the medication you're taking. The main point is that you could get several prescriptions when you're being treated for Alzheimer'sdisease, therefore it's important to be aware of when you feel that one medication is more appropriate than others in your situation.

Experimental Drugs?

What is it they are trying to accomplish?

As we aren't able to give names (there's more than we can list currently) In this article, we'll take you through the most recent research on the experimental Alzheimer's medications. The Alzheimer's drugs that are being tested are looking to boost the creation of acetylcholine within the brain.

If you're not sure what acetylcholine means but don't fret it's an essential chemical found in the brain that is destroyed by Alzheimer's disease. In order to increase the production of this chemical, these medications might be able fight off some of the effects of AD and possibly offer some options for recovery.

The drugs will be considered experimental up to the time that Food and Drug Administration (the FDA) allows their use for the general public. The main point is that scientists are seeking for ways to combat Alzheimer's any way they can. And at present, it appears similar to combating those symptoms as well as slowing the progression of disease while searching for the cure.

About 60% of people notice a reverse of the damage to their brains. the injury must be relatively recent in order for that result to be seen. There's a chance to be hopeful with medications however there's no miracle. Remember that when you consider the objectives of medications, since they're there to ensure all your family members and friends are as comfortable and as content as they can be and give you as much freedom from being affected by Alzheimer's disease as it is possible.

This is the reason this guide is focused on preventing Alzheimer's. When you've been diagnosed with Alzheimer's it is possible to do ways to control it, however, it's not at the same level of freedom as without it. Many of our chapters provide advice that might appear unimportant at this point however they could be more important in the battle against Alzheimer's disease.

Non-Steroidal Anti-Inflammatory Medications (NSAIDs)

What do they mean?

These are your typical Advil, Aleve, Motrin, Tylenol, your over the prescription painkillers.

How do they work?

NSAIDs are most effective when taken in small doses. The majority of Alzheimer's patients are taking 175mg to 500mg or less each day, based on the NSAID being administered at the moment.

What is the reason they do what they do?

Research has shown that NSAIDs are associated with improved performances on cognitive tests in patients with Alzheimer's disease, substantially superior to those taking the drug in a dose that is not sufficient or excessively taking the NSAID dose.

If taken correctly When taken correctly, NSAIDs appear to aid Alzheimer's patients keep some cognitive ability they could lose in the future.

What are the possible side adverse effects?

The adverse effects of NSAIDs are generally minor, primarily focusing upon stomach irritation. The main risk with NSAIDs is the long-term use or excessive doses, since this is linked to bleeding from the stomach kidney failure, stomach bleeding, and other serious side effects.

What time do they call them in?

NSAIDs are a very popular class of drugs used to treat the early signs of Alzheimer's. This is due to the fact that they have experienced great success in treating less severe forms of damage within the brain.

A particular study, conducted in mice, revealed the decrease in beta amyloid, which is a component of the plaque the hallmark of Alzheimer's. The theory is that the beta amyloid part of plaque could be linked to the beginning of the damage. This is because mice that were receiving NSAIDs had not experienced any increases in the amount of plaque.

However they do not actually address the damage to the brain resulted by the Alzheimer's. Alzheimer's disease is still developing, NSAIDs have just been linked with an earlier onset of symptoms.

Prevention, not Treatment

The sad truth about Alzheimer's is that when you're diagnosed, you're aware of what's ahead. The treatment and medication options can help to delay the development of the disease However, in the end, Alzheimer's will be a traumatic injury to it to the point where you are unable to comprehend fundamental concepts.

It's a scary thought I can understand the fear. The idea of having Alzheimer's disease is a source of fear for many when they think of getting older and that's a good thing. The point of this article is not to make you feel scared however, to urge you to contact your family members and go to the library together, picking some resources about what's to come and the best way to understand the disease. We've compiled a list in the appendix based on this guideline to help you get going.

The principal purpose in this article is simply to present my findings about how to stop Alzheimer's. No matter if you're suffering from Alzheimer's or it is a part of the family or may know someone who suffers from it You should take steps for ways to safeguard your family and yourself from its harmful effects.

Do not believe that there's no hope for you even if it is a part of your family, be aware of the less-than-perfect connection between the family history of your parents and Alzheimer's. This guide will give you strategies and suggestions to improve your choices in lifestyle and prepare your body with the tools to fight Alzheimer's.

It is important to note that even if you are diagnosed with Alzheimer's disease, you can try to slow the progression of the symptoms by following the suggestions included in this guide. While you can predict the direction your mind is likely to take you, you do not have any idea of when it will arrive.

Some may think it's too far, but for the ones who are reading this now, there are steps that need to be taken to safeguard yourself and those you love. The steps are about maintaining a sharp mind, regardless of what you're thinking you can accomplish this!

There are natural methods Too!

We're done with explanations. You've read about the causes of Alzheimer's disease, what it can do to your body, as well as the treatments that are used to combat it. Now , it's time to dig into what you're really looking for: the study of the prevention of Alzheimer's disease.

From this chapter I will concentrate on only presenting the tried and tested methods to stop Alzheimer's. Each of them is centered on the health of your brain as well as the well-being that your body. If you keep your body and mind well-maintained, we'll take every step to provide you with protections against Alzheimer's disease, so that, even if you do develop it, you'll be able to see a delay in its beginning (at at the very minimum) and possibly there will be no onset!

What kind of strategies will we look at?

Let's talk about the most common. In the beginning, I will talk about the drugs. There are two principal drugs that can delay the onset of Alzheimer's disease. beginning, and they are known as Aricept or Cognac. Both of these medications have been accepted by the FDA and are extensively utilized as cholinesterase inhibiters.

You might be wondering what's so special is acetylcholine. Remember, acetylcholine is the neurotransmitter we've talked about so much. What makes acetylcholine so vital is its ability to block cholinesterase once it's correctly broken down. The medicines we've discussed in the previous paragraphs are designed to do just this, as do the treatment options in this guide.

The distinction in this article is the fact that it will help you see the breakdown of acetylcholine in a natural way.

I will briefly mention the medications and I do so as I realize that you would like to be aware of the names of medicines the guide is built on. I have identified these drugs to understand the underlying cause of what we're trying to accomplish to prevent and delay the development of Alzheimer's, which is to block cholinesterase.

I will provide you with the best herbs, minerals and vitamins that you should include in your daily diet. I will demonstrate things which you are able to do to maintain your brain alert. I'll even give you exercises that will help on the fight against Alzheimer's. And, most importantly? I will inform you each stage of my journey on the reasons I am doing these things and why these things so crucial to you.

Do not rush out to buy acetylcholine supplements now. Take a look at the chapters that follow. I will discuss a variety of minerals, herbs and vitamins that aid in enhancing the body's capacity to perform this task. I will also go over each step of the process to explain why these elements are crucial to you, in order that you can take your food choices with a sense of understanding and willpower.

Finally, I'd like to know how to most effectively use this chapter. I've listed the treatments according to their classifications. As an example, many of vitamins are antioxidants which is why we'll be discussing antioxidants. Building your immune system can be an excellent way to remain healthy, so we'll be talking on the nutrients that aid in this. And the list goes on. Through breaking it down by the category, I've made this guide simpler to refer back to whenever you're struggling with certain aspects of your diet.

For instance, if you're suffering from free radicals, you'll need to visit the section on antioxidants in this article, while in the event that you're weak from illness, you might want to build the immune system.

The fact of education an important tool to keep your brain active and the more you are aware of ways to fight Alzheimer's disease the better you'll be at battling it. This guide will give you a wealth of information that is arranged in the most easy to comprehend ways that are possible, and with a way that allows you to go back to previous chapters.

You can revisit the charts on the next pages at any point. I've laid them out for you to see your choices and there are many. Do not expect to know them all.

Ready? Let's go.

Antioxidants

What are they doing?

To comprehend what antioxidants can help you You must be aware of the free radical cell. Our body comprised by millions of cell. Each of which is composed of the atoms. I know I'm sure however, it's just an introduction to science.

The thing you should be aware of is that there are certain cells that don't have a concern for the body. These are called free radical cells and if they are left unchallenged they'll spread themselves across the body, creating destruction everywhere they are. This can have a negative effect upon the wellbeing and health of various organs and bodily functions but the main issue we're looking at right now is the impact of the

174

brain. When free radicals attack your brain area, they start to destroy the neurons and weaken the connections ones that your brain needs to efficiently process the information it receives.

This can lead to issues like memories being lost, tremors, and eventually the frightening loss of ability to connect the most basic ideas.

As you might have guessed already, antioxidants combat Free radicals. They specifically target them before further damage is caused.

Where can we find them?

It is possible to get antioxidants through your diet. Many foods contain antioxidants naturally particularly organic ones as well as whole grain.

There are also some of them from your body however, if you don't increase these levels naturally as you get older you'll notice they're not helping as much (because there aren't as many as they used to be).

Alpha Lipoic Acid (ALA)

What are the implications?

Alpha Lipoic Acid is a particular antioxidant. We've covered antioxidants and their role above, they fight the free radical cell.

What differentiates ALA from the others is its capacity to act not just as an antioxidantbut to stimulate the growth of other antioxidants and stimulate glutathione.

Glutathione is a powerful antioxidant that can reverse the damage caused by nerves and boost the defense of cells in one go. Researchers have been enthralled by ALA due to this reason. it boosts glutathione (which could help in reducing damage to nerves) as well as other antioxidants (only providing a double effects you're getting).

With the advancement of research, we are now able to see that ALA is remarkable not just because of its link to damaged nerves that can be reversed however, it also has a potential link to improve memory. Researchers who are who are behind these researches are exuberant, and with great reason. ALA could be the most exciting discovery of the future!

Where do you look for it?

Your body produces naturally alpha Lipoic acid however, not in amounts enough to create an impact on the antioxidant levels. Where do you go to increase your levels? It's all in the diet. ALA is found in spinach, liver and yeast.

Acetyl-L-Carnitine (ALC)

What is its purpose?

ALC can be described as an antioxidant. We've talked about this numerous times and antioxidants are fantastic to prevent Alzheimer's as well as for your health due to the fact that they stop the growth of free radical cells and assist your body to fight existing ones.

Aside from its antioxidant benefits, ALC also stimulates acetylcholine in the brain. Acetylcholine is the neurotransmitter that causes can be used to combat Alzheimer's and any supplementation which boosts its supply of it should be considered extremely beneficial for fighting the fight to prevent and slow down the development of Alzheimer's. ALC accomplishes this by keeping healthy levels of acetylcholine within the brain.

ALC is also used worldwide to treat neurodegenerative conditions due to its capacity to prevent brain damage. It is probably because of its ability to increase acetylcholine levels, but regardless, we know that it does work.

A clinical study looked at over 500 Alzheimer's and dementia patients. The study discovered that

ALC was able to in repairing some damage to the brain that had occurred and slow the decline in memory. In addition, it aid in improving communication and concentration levels during the study.

Conclusion

It is evident that we need to be educated about the possibilities and options of the homeopathic, non-invasive Alzheimer's treatment. The most important thing is to be aware that the loss of memory and cognitive degeneration isn't an inevitable aspect of aging, however, it is caused by poor nutrition physical and emotional insomnia, stress and social isolation. In lieu of treating condition lifestyle changes have led to great success in reducing the likelihood of suffering from Alzheimer's disease. They have also succeeded in encouraging the brain combat the symptoms by creating new neural pathways and promoting the growth of the brain. Even if plaques and knots are beginning to appear with the proper lifestyle changes and the right exercises can ease signs of the disease , and individuals can live an active, healthy life. In the same way those with a low risk of developing Alzheimer's disease can greatly benefit from small changes and adding exercises into their routine. Everyone gets benefit from the development of their brains.

The idea of afflicting Alzheimer's disease with the inevitable decline of mental health is false and sets people up for the worst instead of encouraging individuals to make adjustments and engage in exercises. There is more control we have over our health and brain function than we realize - a lot of easy exercises have proved to be extremely efficient, especially in preventing or slowing the progress in the course of disease. Nutrition also has a greater impact than we think and it is important to be aware of what food items we consume regularly as they play a significant influence on how we think.

It is crucial to be aware of false statements of health experts who promote a low cholesterol diet, low fat and to instead lower sugars and other simple carbs , while also incorporating a wide range of food high in omega-3s and vitamins or taking supplements. Although the diagnosis of Alzheimer's disease is difficult to manage but the despair and hopelessness associated with the illness prevent people from taking the needed actions to combat it. Instead, we must be motivated and encourage others to improve their the health of their brains and encourage development in every way that is possible.

Thank you for buying this book. It is my wish that it will aid people in dealing with a horrible disease.

CPSIA information can be obtained
at www.ICGtesting.com
Printed in the USA
BVHW060850310522
638499BV00015B/285

9 781774 854648